P N Nightingale

Neurotrauma

Treatment, Rehabilitation, and Related Issues

No. 1

Neurotrauma

Treatment, Rehabilitation, and Related Issues

No. 1

Edited by
Michael E. Miner, *M.D., Ph.D.*
Associate Professor and Director
Division of Neurosurgery
University of Texas Medical School at Houston
Houston, Texas

Karen A. Wagner, *Ph.D.*
Coordinator of Research
Division of Neurosurgery
University of Texas Medical School at Houston
Houston, Texas

with 28 contributing authors

Butterworths
Boston London Durban Singapore Sydney Toronto Wellington

Every effort has been made to ensure that the drug dosage schedules within this text are accurate and conform to standards accepted at time of publication. However, as treatment recommendations vary in the light of continuing research and clinical experience, the reader is advised to verify drug dosage schedules herein with information found on product information sheets. This is especially true in cases of new or infrequently used drugs.

Library of Congress Cataloging-in-Publication Data

Main entry under title:

Neurotrauma: treatment, rehabilitation, and related issues.

   Proceedings of the First Houston Conference on
Neurotrauma, held in May 1984.
   Includes bibliographies and index.
   1. Head—Wounds and injuries—Congresses.
2. Brain—Wounds and injuries—Complications and
sequelae—Congresses.   3. Head—Wounds and injuries—
Patients—Rehabilitation—Congresses.   I. Miner,
Michael E.   II. Wagner, Karen A.   III. Houston
Conference on Neurotrauma (1st : 1984) [DNLM:
1. Evoked Potentials—congresses.   2. Head Injuries—
rehabilitation—congresses.   3. Head Injuries—therapy—
congresses.   WE 706 N494 1984]
RD521.N48   1986   617'.48044   86–953
ISBN 0–409–95167–6

Butterworths
80 Montvale Avenue
Stoneham, MA 02180

10   9   8   7   6   5   4   3   2   1

Printed in the United States of America

Contents

Contributing Authors

Steven J. Allen, M.D.
Clinical Instructor, Department of Anesthesiology, University of Texas Medical School at Houston, Texas

Guy L. Clifton, M.D.
Assistant Professor of Neurosurgery, Baylor College of Medicine, Houston, Texas

D. Nathan Cope, M.D.
Assistant Professor and Chief, Division of Rehabilitation Medicine, Santa Clara Valley Medical Center, San Jose, California

Julio Cruz, M.D.
Visiting Assistant Professor of Neurosurgery, University of Texas Medical School at Houston, Texas

Michael F. Domurat, M.D.
Resident in Anesthesiology, Albert Einstein College of Medicine, Bronx, New York

Howard M. Eisenberg, M.D.
Professor and Chief, Division of Neurosurgery, University of Texas Medical Branch at Galveston, Texas

H. Tristram Engelhardt, Jr., Ph.D., M.D.
Professor of Medicine and of Community Medicine and Member, Center for Ethics, Medicine, and Public Issues, Baylor College of Medicine, Houston, Texas

Linda Ewing-Cobbs, Ph.D.
Research Associate, Department of Psychiatry and Behavioral Sciences, University of Texas Medical School at Houston, Texas

Jack M. Fletcher, Ph.D.
Chief, Developmental Neuropsychology Section, Texas Research Institute of Mental Sciences, Houston, Texas

Ralph F. Frankowski, Ph.D.
Professor of Biometry, University of Texas School of Public Health, Houston, Texas

Elizabeth A.M. Frost, M.D.
Professor of Anesthesiology, Albert Einstein College of Medicine, Bronx, New York

James W. Hall III, Ph.D.
Associate Professor and Chief of Audiology, Department of Otolaryngology—Head and Neck Surgery, University of Texas Medical School at Houston, Texas

Karyl M. Hall, Ph.D.
Project Administrator/Coordinator, Northern California Regional Spinal Injury System, San Jose, California

Stanley F. Handel, M.D.
Adjunct Professor of Epidemiology, University of Texas School of Public Health, Houston, Texas

Tessa Hart, Ph.D.
Director of Research, Department of Neuropsychology, Medical Center Del Oro Hospital, Houston, Texas

Mary Ellen Hayden, Ph.D.
Director of Neuropsychology, Medical Center Del Oro Hospital, Houston, Texas

Dennis R. Kopaniky, M.D., Ph.D.
Assistant Professor of Neurosurgery, University of Texas Medical School at Houston, Texas

Harvey S. Levin, Ph.D.
Professor of Neurosurgery, University of Texas Medical School at Galveston, Texas

Judy R. Makey-Hargadine, M.D.
Assistant Professor of Neurosurgery, University of Texas Medical School at Houston, Texas

Michael E. Miner, M.D., Ph.D.
Associate Professor and Director, Division of Neurosurgery, University of Texas Medical School at Houston, Texas

H. Gustav Mueller, Ph.D.
Supervisor, Audiology Section, Army Audiology and Speech Center, Walter Reed Army Medical Center, Washington, D.C.

Daniel P. Perales, M.P.H.
Program Manager, Houston-Galveston Injury Prevention Group

Maurice Rappaport, M.D. Ph.D.
Academic Administrator, University of California at San Francisco, and Research Department, University of California Brain Function Lab, Agnews State Hospital, San Jose, California

Claudia S. Robertson, M.D.
Assistant Professor, Department of Neurosurgery, Baylor College of Medicine, Houston, Texas

Andres M. Salazar, M.D.
Director, Vietnam Head Injury Study, Walter Reed Army Medical Center, Washington, D.C.

Roy K. Sedge, Ph.D.
Director, Army Audiology and Speech Center, Walter Reed Army Medical Center, Washington, D.C.

Karen A. Wagner, Ph.D.
Coordinator of Research, Division of Neurosurgery, University of Texas Medical School at Houston, Texas

L. James Willmore, M.D.
Associate Professor of Neurology, University of Texas Medical School at Houston, Texas

Preface

Over the past twenty years a sophisticated, well-organized approach to the rapid resuscitation of trauma victims has emerged. Many patients who in the past would not have survived their injury are now saved, and cases that once involved only the acute care team today call upon the skills of a spectrum of health professionals who will play a role in restoring patients to their fullest functional level in the aftermath of injury. What happens to the trauma patient at each stage of management is influenced by what occurred before and in turn affects what will follow. Yet we, as health professionals, tend to focus on our own segment of patient care and are often poorly informed about our colleagues' roles.

With more and more of our medical resources required to treat an injury victim, a group of us in Houston began to consider what avenues for discussion and learning were available to professionals working with patients who have sustained trauma to the central nervous system. We concluded that no satisfactory forum existed for examining the full range of issues pertinent to CNS trauma from an advanced-level, multidisciplinary perspective. The First Houston Conference on Neurotrauma, from which this volume emanates, was convened to answer this perceived need. The conference was organized to bring together professionals involved in the entire spectrum of study and management of head injury, from acute resuscitation to intensive care, medical and surgical management, rehabilitation, and reintegration into the community.

The conference was planned as the first of a series of annual meetings from which books will be published expanding in depth on selected presentations. Each volume will address a range of treatment, rehabilitation, and other pertinent issues that we consider particularly timely; this first volume, for example, features a section on the use of evoked responses for assessing parameters of morbidity or recovery. The response to this approach has been gratifying and we plan to proceed with the same basic format in the future. The diversity of topics and wide range of interests of the many specialists working on new, innovative, and challenging clinical and laboratory investigations in the broad area of head injury research makes a multidisciplinary approach continually appealing.

We are indebted to Ms. Anne Brown, Mr. Randy Johnson, Dr. Daniel Morrison, and Dr. Mary Ellen Hayden of the Medical Center Del Oro Hospital and Dr. Dennis Kopaniky, Ms. Gloria Horner, and Ms. Lou Esposito of the University of Texas, Houston, for their help in planning the conference and for their support in the preparation of this book.

M.E.M.
K.A.W.

Neurotrauma

*Treatment, Rehabilitation,
and Related Issues*

No. 1

Chapter 1

The Demography of Head Injury in the United States

Ralph F. Frankowski

Accidents, homicide, and suicide are major determinants of mortality in the United States. In 1980 these three causes of death were responsible for a total of nearly 160,000 deaths. About two-thirds of the total number of fatal injuries were caused by accidents, primarily motor vehicle accidents. The remaining one-third were accounted for by homicide and suicide, in nearly equal proportions. One of every twelve deaths in the United States in 1980 resulted from injuries that were unintentional or deliberate in occurrence [1].

Injury is the major cause of death for the young. It is the leading cause of death for persons aged 1 to 44 years, whether black or white, male or female [1]. As a result, injury robs society of persons entering their most productive years and is the leading cause of productive years of life lost for the population of the United States, exceeding diseases of the heart, malignant neoplasms, and cerebrovascular diseases [2].

Estimates of morbidity due to injury are equally high. The National Health Interview Survey estimated that in 1981 nearly 70 million persons, one-third of the total population of the United States, sustained injuries that involved at least 1 day of restricted activity or required medical attendance [3]. The National Hospital Discharge Survey reported that injuries ranked fifth in 1980 as the primary diagnosis among all patients discharged from nonfederal hospitals, accounting for 3.6 million hospital discharges in 1980 [4]. There are about twenty hospital discharges for injury for each death due to injury, a ratio that illustrates the ubiquitous nature of intentional and unintentional injury in the United States.

The growing recognition of the relationship between injuries and health and the exceptional demand that injuries place on the medical care system have prompted population studies of specific life-threatening injuries in order to understand their causes, sequelae, and the options available to reduce the magnitude of the problem. Among life-threatening injuries, few are feared more than brain injury. Injury to the brain caused by mechanical energy often results in death, and lesser injury to the brain is well recognized for its potential

1

to cause transient or irreversible neurological, neuropsychological, and functional impairments [5].

This chapter reviews the recent major findings on the occurrence of head and brain injuries in defined populations. The chapter focuses on the demography and epidemiology of head and brain injury, the immediate causes of such injuries, the populations most severely affected, and the strategies available for the control and prevention of brain injury.

HEAD INJURY AS A CAUSE OF DEATH IN THE UNITED STATES

The medical information that is recorded on death certificates is the basis for the tabulation of national cause of death statistics. These statistics are based solely on the determination of the underlying cause of death. For injuries, the underlying cause of death refers to the circumstances of the accident or violence that produced the fatal injury. The underlying cause of death is selected in accordance with the procedures and rules prescribed by the International Classification of Diseases, adapted for use in the United States (ICDA) [6].

For deaths due to injuries, the ICDA provides a dual classification. Injury deaths are assigned an E code, describing the external cause of the fatal injury, and an N code, indicating the nature (pathology) of the injury. By custom, national cause of death statistics for injuries are tabulated only by the E codes that describe the circumstances or violence that produced the fatal injury. Thus, the annual number of deaths and the population risks of death due to brain or head injury in the United States is not routinely reported.

In spring 1984, the National Center for Health Statistics published a landmark national report [7]. This report tabulated for the first time the nature of injury codes recorded for all deaths occurring in a single year, 1978. The nature of injury codes (N850–N854) for intracranial injury, excluding skull fracture, appeared for 24% of all deaths due to injury for the United States in 1978. Although the national data have not been fully reviewed for their accuracy and completeness, it is fairly safe to infer that at least one of every four fatal injuries that occurred in the United States in 1978 involved a significant intracranial injury. About 28% of all deaths with mention of intracranial injury (excluding those with skull fracture) occurred to persons aged 15 to 24 years. Intracranial injuries were reported to cause more deaths for males than for females by a ratio of 3:1 [7].

Detailed information from national death certificate tabulations on the population risk of death from head injury and its demographic correlates is extremely limited. However, during the 1970s, specialized research studies on the risk of fatal head injuries have been conducted for a variety of populations, and these studies can be pieced together to derive a limited sketch of the population risks of fatal head injuries in the United States.

The first community-based study of the incidence, causes, and secular trends of head trauma was published by Annegers et al [8]. Records in the Mayo Clinic linkage system were reviewed to identify the incidence of head trauma among residents of Olmsted County, Minnesota, for the time period 1935 to 1974. All death certificates and autopsy protocols of Olmsted County residents were also reviewed. Head trauma was defined as an injury with evidence of presumed brain involvement, as manifested by intracranial injury, loss of consciousness, posttraumatic amnesia, or skull fracture. Fatal head injuries were restricted to deaths occurring within 28 days of the initial injury. The average age-adjusted rate of fatal head injuries for the population of Olmsted County, during the decade 1965 to 1974, was 22 head injury deaths per 100,000 population.

Klauber et al [9] reported a prospective study of all deaths from head injury and all patients admitted to hospitals with a diagnosis of head injury in San Diego County, California, during 1978. Fatal head injuries were defined by selected ICDA codes that identified individuals whose head injury resulted in intracranial injury, skull fracture, coma, amnesia, neurologic deficit, or seizures but excluded those with head lacerations or bruises to the head. Gunshot wounds were excluded by the design of the prospective study. The overall head injury mortality (excluding gunshot) for San Diego County in 1978 was estimated at 22.3 deaths per 100,000 population.

In 1981 a collaborative survey of head injury mortality was conducted in three major metropolitan populations as part of the National Institutes of Health–National Institute of Neurological, Communicative Disorders, and Stroke Program for the establishment of comprehensive treatment and research centers for central nervous system injury [10]. The study populations were those of Bronx County, New York; Harris County, Texas; and San Diego County, California. Fatal head injuries were defined by the ICDA rubrics of skull fractures and intracranial injuries. Deaths were ascertained from among all deaths due to accidents, suicides, and homicides using death certificates, autopsy reports, and hospital records. All head injury deaths recorded for residents of each study county for the calendar year 1980 were included. Head injury mortality ranged from 27 per 100,000 population (Bronx County) to 32 per 100,000 population (Harris County).

A third study of the population of San Diego County, California, was conducted by Kraus et al [11] to determine the incidence of acute brain injury and serious impairment among residents for 1981. Brain injury was defined as physical damage to, or functional impairment of, the cranial contents from acute mechanical energy exchange. This definition included all intracranial injuries and injuries to the brain stem extending to the level of the first cervical vertebra. All persons with autopsy evidence of brain injury sustained in 1981 were included. Excluded were skull fractures or soft tissue damage without concurrent brain injury. The overall brain injury mortality rate, from all traumatic causes, for the 1981 population of San Diego County was estimated at 30 deaths per 100,000 population.

The most recent report on mortality rates from head trauma comes from

Whitman and co-workers [12] in a study of the incidence of head trauma in two small, socioeconomically different Chicago-area communities: one located in the inner city of Chicago, the other in the city of Evanston, a Chicago suburb. Cases were ascertained by hospital ICDA rubrics for intracranial injuries with the requirement that the injury had onset within 7 days prior to hospitalization and included one or more of the following: (1) a blow to the head, (2) a blow to the face accompanied by loss of consciousness, (3) a laceration of scalp or forehead. Head injury deaths of the residents of the two communities were determined by neurologic review of the records of the county medical examiner. Mortality rates from head injury were 32 for the inner city Chicago community and 13 per 100,000 for Evanston.

The results of these four studies of head injury as a cause of death suggest that head injury mortality rates vary considerably among communities in the United States. The reported annual number of deaths due to head injury varies from 13 per 100,000 population for the city of Evanston, Illinois, to 32 per 100,000 population for Harris County, Texas, and the inner city community of Chicago. This remarkable variation in injury death results from the influence and interplay of three major factors: (1) the size and demographic composition of the communities, (2) the extent of exposure within each community to the causes of fatal injuries, and (3) study differences in case ascertainment and reporting procedures. If some of the major demographic, exposure, and reporting features are controlled, the variation of head injury mortality rates in the types of populations studied is consistent, plausible, and informative of the likely national situation.

Table 1.1 presents data on head injury mortality of males and females from each of the populations reported in the selected studies. The table demonstrates that head injury mortality is substantially higher in males than in females. The ratios of male to female mortality range from 2.2 to 4.6. Female head injury mortality is uniformly low and shows little variation among the populations while male mortality varies widely among the populations.

Population age-specific head injury mortality rates typically show a bimodal appearance (Figure 1.1). Peak head injury mortality occurs at 15 to 24 and over 70 years of age. Male and female head injury mortality is similar to the age of 15, but then male mortality increases rapidly and exceeds female mortality at least threefold throughout adult life [8,10,11]. The most extreme differences in male and female mortality occur among young adults and the elderly [8,10,11,12,13]. Age- and sex-specific patterns of head injury mortality vary among the populations in proportion to the extent and exposure of the populations to the causes of fatal injuries.

Table 1.2 presents the percentage distribution of the causes of fatal head injuries from the selected studies. Transportation injuries and gunshot wounds are the leading causes of fatal injuries in each population. Overall, transportation and gunshot injuries account for about three of every four fatal head injuries. In the crowded and largely poor populations of Bronx County and

Table 1.1 Head Injury Mortality as Reported in Selected Studies, by Sex per 100,000 Population per Year

Population and Year	Source	Number of Deaths per 100,000 Population		Male/Female Ratio
		Male	Female	
Olmsted County, Minn. (1965–1974)	[8]	35	10	3.5
San Diego County, Calif. (1978)	[9]	32[a]	12[a]	2.7
Bronx County, N.Y. (1980)	[10]	48	12	4
Harris County, Tex. (1980)	[10]	51	13	3.9
San Diego County, Calif. (1980)	[10]	42	11	3.8
Inner City Chicago, Ill. (1980)	[12]	55	12	4.6
Evanston, Ill. (1980)	[12]			
Black population		27	12	2.2
White population		16	7	2.3
San Diego County, Calif. (1981)	[11]	45	10	4.5

[a]Rates exclude head injury deaths due to gunshot.

inner city Chicago, more than half of all fatal injuries are due to gunshot wounds or blunt-instrument trauma assault, while in the more affluent and dispersed county populations, transportation injuries account for nearly half of all fatal head injuries.

Gunshot wounds present an interesting contrast among the populations reported in Table 1.2. In Bronx County and inner city Chicago, 96% of the fatal gunshot wounds were the result of interpersonal violence [10,12]. In Harris County, Texas, where the percentage (44%) of fatal gunshot wounds exceeds the percentage (40%) of fatal gunshot wounds in the Bronx, about 50% of the fatal gunshot wounds were self-inflicted [10]. There is also an interesting association between the data presented in Tables 1.1 and 1.2. An almost linear relation exists between the male head injury death rates and the percentages of fatal head injury deaths due to gunshot. This implies that the proportion of fatal head injury gunshot wounds is an excellent predictor of total male head injury mortality. Conversely, female head injury mortality varies little with the levels of gunshot mortality among the populations. Thus, it can be inferred from the current data that fatal head injury due to gunshot is essentially a male-dominant affliction.

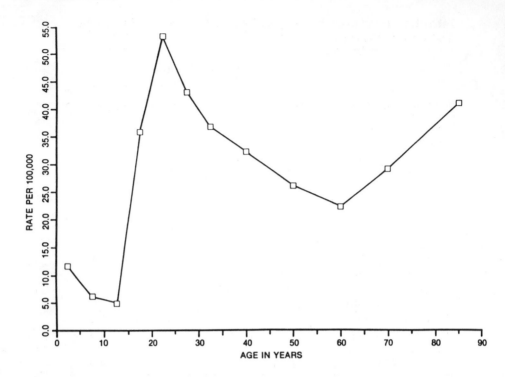

Figure 1.1   1980 age-specific death rates for head injury for the combined populations of Bronx County, N.Y., Harris County, Tex., and San Diego County, Calif.

Falls are the third leading cause of fatal head injuries, averaging about 10% as a cause of death among the reported studies (Table 1.2). Falls affect the very young and the elderly most frequently [8].

Racial and ethnic differentials for head injury mortality have been reported in detail for the population of Bronx County, New York [13]. The age-adjusted incidence of head injury mortality for the black and Hispanic populations exceeded the head injury mortality of the white population by ratios of 1.8 and 1.5 respectively. The higher relative risks for the minority populations were due to excess male head injury deaths caused by violence. Whitman, in his study of Evanston, Illinois, reported similar findings, with a relative risk of head injury mortality of 1.7 for the black population [12]. Whitman also observed substantial mortality differences between the black populations of the inner city and of the suburban areas. The inner city black population experienced head injury mortality at a rate three times the rate of the suburban black population as a result of deaths due to interpersonal violence. In minority populations, as in the white populations, head injury mortality is concentrated among males. In the black, Hispanic, and white female populations of Bronx

Table 1.2 Percent Distribution of Fatal Head Injuries from Selected Studies, by Major Categories of External Causes

| Population and Year | Source | N^a | External Cause | | | | | |
			Transportation	Falls	Assault	Gunshot	Other
Olmsted County, Minn. (1934–1974)	[8]	446	53%	14%	1%	20%	12%
Bronx County, N.Y. (1980)	[10]	313	20	18	15	40	7
Harris County, Tex. (1980)	[10]	758	44	5	4	44	3
San Diego County, Calif. (1980)	[10]	476	49	15	5	28	3
Inner City Chicago, Ill. (1979)	[12]	45	22	NR	13	56	9

[a]Total number of head injury deaths.
NR = not reported.

County, New York, the incidence of death due to head injury was less than 6 per 100,000 population for all causes, including violence [13].

Table 1.3 presents data on the place of death of the fatal head injuries as reported in the selected studies. At least two-thirds of all head injury deaths occurred prior to hospital inpatient care. This is a distinctive feature of head injury mortality that reveals its devastating and rapid course. In populations where substantial numbers of gunshot wounds were reported, such as Bronx County, New York, and Harris County, Texas, nearly 3 of every 4 head injury deaths occurred prior to hospital inpatient care. A similar finding was reported by the Emergency Medical Services System of Hudson Valley, New York [14]. Of 211 consecutive brain injury deaths, 156 (73.9%) occurred at the scene, on hospital arrival, or in a hospital emergency room. The Hudson Valley survey reported two-thirds of all brain injury deaths as immediate deaths or deaths on arrival (DOA). Postmortem studies concluded that none of the DOA cases was considered preventable by more rapid transport or exceptional emergency medical services treatment [14].

The only data on secular trends in head injury mortality in the United States come from the population study of Olmsted County for the period 1935 to 1974. Over this time period the age-adjusted head injury death rate of 22 per 100,000 population remained constant [8].

In summary, the combined data from the selected studies suggest that the head injury death rate in the United States is 20 to 30 head injury deaths per 100,000 population. Peak mortality, of at least twice the overall rate, is likely among young adults and the elderly population. Males are at three to four times the risk of females to sustain a lethal head injury, except among the very young where the mortality rates for both sexes are about equal. Transportation injuries, gunshot wounds, and falls account for at least 75% of

Table 1.3 Relative Frequency of Hospital and Nonhospital Head Injury Deaths as Reported in Selected Studies

Population and Year	Source	Number of Deaths	Percent Hospital	Percent Nonhospital[a]
Bronx County, N.Y. (1980)	[10]	328	25.3%	74.7%
Harris County, Tex. (1980)	[10]	758	26.6	73.4
Chicago area[b] (1980)	[12]	54	33.3	66.7
San Diego County, Calif. (1981)	[11]	562	31.3	68.7

[a]Includes persons who died immediately at the scene or who were pronounced dead at a hospital emergency room.
[b]Deaths from the inner city Chicago community and Evanston, Ill., are combined in this category.

all fatal head injuries. Approximately two-thirds of all injury deaths are non-hospital deaths, most of which are likely to be immediate deaths.

INCIDENCE STUDIES OF HEAD AND BRAIN INJURY

Deaths due to head injury are a reliable guide to the most extreme effect of head injury but offer little indication of the extent of population morbidity due to head and brain injury. Morbidity and mortality population risks can be jointly estimated by incidence studies of the occurrence of head injury in defined populations. The incidence of head or brain injury refers to the number of new cases of head or brain injury that occur per year in a population. Incidence cases are restricted to those ascertained from hospitals or records of medical examiners.

Since 1974, seven incidence studies of head injury have been conducted for various populations of the United States [8,9,11,12,13,18,19]. Much of the published data are limited by the usual problems of incidence surveys. No two studies used identical definitions of head injury, although all had a stated objective to estimate the incidence of brain injury for the defined populations. The methodological problem in ascertaining all cases of brain injury in a population, for all levels of severity, is that brain injury can occur with only subtle signs and symptoms that are often difficult to uncover in routine hospital records. Further, Jennett has argued that there can be no absolute criteria for brain injury since the scalp, skull, and brain can each be injured without involvement of the other [15]. Thus, the studies have varied widely in their approaches to the ascertainment of actual and presumed brain injury. At a minimum, all studies followed Jennett's precept that actual or potential brain injury ascertainment requires knowledge of a blow to the head and altered consciousness [16], but they were often limited by the information available in hospital medical records. Comparisons are further limited by the variety of methods used for case ascertainment and inclusion. Studies differed in their inclusion of nonhospital fatal injuries, the residency determination of cases, and the inclusion of nonhospitalized but medically treated cases. These and other methodologic differences among the studies are discussed elsewhere [17].

Table 1.4 presents the incidence rates per 100,000 population of head or brain injury as reported in the seven incidence studies [19], and Table 1.5 presents incidence ratios by sex and race. Although it is not possible to make sharp comparisons among populations, a few general conclusions about the incidence of head injury appear possible. The incidence rates are surprisingly similar when examined by the racial and ethnic characteristics of the populations. White or predominantly white populations show incidence in the range of 180 to 230 head or brain injuries per 100,000 population. The 1978 San Diego County survey overestimated incidence because of the inclusion of head injuries to nonresidents and the use of provisional estimates of the population

Table 1.4 Incidence Rates of Head Injury as Reported in Selected Studies per 100,000 Population per Year

Population, Year, and Source	Case-finding Sources	Case-finding Criteria	Incidence
U.S. population (1974) [19]	Hospital inpatient admissions, discharges, and deaths	Search of selected ICD codes[c]	200
Olmsted County, Minn. (1965–1974) [8]	Hospital inpatient admissions, emergency room visits, outpatient exams, home visits, hospital and nonhospital death records	Concussion with loss of consciousness, posttraumatic amnesia, neurologic signs of brain injury, skull fracture	193
San Diego County, Calif. (1978) [9]	Hospital inpatient admissions,[a,b] hospital and nonhospital death records[a,b]	Search of selected ICD codes[c]	295
North Central Virginia (1978) [18]	Hospital inpatient admissions and deaths[b]	Loss of consciousness, posttraumatic amnesia, skull fracture	208
Bronx County, N.Y. (1980) [13]	Hospital admissions and discharges, emergency room visits, hospital and nonhospital death records	Loss of consciousness, skull fracture, posttraumatic seizures, neurologic signs of brain injury	249
Evanston, Ill. (1980) Inner City Chicago, Ill. (1980) [12]	Hospital inpatient discharges, hospital and nonhospital death records	Search of selected ICD codes[c]	233 403
San Diego County, Calif. (1981) [11]	Hospital inpatient discharges, emergency room visits, nursing home and extended care records, hospital and nonhospital deaths	Search of selected ICD codes, [c] confirmed brain injury only	180

[a]Excluding gunshot wounds.
[b]Including nonresidents.
[c]Although International Classification of Diseases (ICD) case-finding codes varied among studies, all studies included concussion, skull fracture, and intracranial injuries.

Table 1.5 Ratio of Head Injury Incidence Rates, by Sex and Race, for Selected Studies

Population and Year	Source	Ratio of Incidence	
		Male to Female	Black to White
United States (1974)[a]	[19]	2.1	0.90[b]
Olmsted County, Minn. (1965–1974)	[8]	2.3	Not reported
San Diego County, Calif. (1978)	[9]	1.6	Not reported
North Central Virginia (1978)[a]	[18]	2.1	1.5
Inner City Chicago, Ill. (1979)	[12]	2.5	2.5 Not reported
Evanston, Ill. (1979)	[12]	2.4	2.0
Bronx County, N.Y. (1980)	[13]	2.8	1.3
San Diego County, Calif. (1981)[c]	[11]	2.2	Not reported

[a]Excludes nonhospital deaths.
[b]Nonwhite to white incidence ratio.
[c]Acute brain injuries only.

that later were found to be too low [11]. Conversely, incidence from the National Head and Spinal Cord Injury Survey is underestimated since the survey excluded nonhospital head injury deaths, which occur with a frequency of at least 10 per 100,000 population [19]. However, the combined data suggest an average crude incidence rate of head or brain injury of about 200 to 225 per 100,000 population for the white population of the United States. The reported incidence rates for the minority populations are higher (Table 1.5). However, the minority populations studied are atypical and likely overrepresent violence-prone populations. If averaged across the full spectrum of socioeconomic conditions, incidence rates of head injury for minority populations are likely to be only slightly above white rates [12].

A general bimodal distribution of the age-specific incidence of head injury has been reported by all the selected studies. Peak incidences occur among young adults and the elderly although the degree and extent of bimodality varies with the demographic composition of the population and the distribution of risk factors (causes) within populations. Typically, head injury incidence rates per 100,000 population are about 150 for ages 0 to 4, increase to about 550 for ages 15 to 24, fall gradually to about 160 at age 50, and increase again with age. At age 65 and beyond, the incidence of head injury is approximately 200 per 100,000 population. Males are at about twice the risk of females for sustaining a head injury. Male to female incidence ratios vary by age, cause, and severity, but male incidence typically exceeds female incidence for all causes [11]. At the ages of 15 to 24, males are about three times more likely to experience a head injury than females. In the 1981 study of San Diego County, nearly 70% of all acute brain injuries occurred to males [11]. Differences in male and female incidence appear in the first decade of life [8,11,12,13,18], suggesting that young males and females differ not only in the degrees of risk to head injury but also in the kinds of risks.

Traffic and transportation accidents are the leading cause of head injuries, explaining one-third to one-half of hospitalized injuries (Table 1.6). Falls are the second leading cause, accounting for 20 to 30% of all head injuries. Interpersonal violence explains 7 to 40% of all incident cases, but its intensity varies significantly among the selected populations. In Bronx County and inner city Chicago, violence and transportation accidents are almost equal causes of all head injuries.

The severity of head injuries is reported in three of the population studies: Olmsted County, Evanston and inner city Chicago, and the 1981 San Diego County survey [8,11,12]. In each of these studies, trivial and mild head injuries accounted for 60 to 80% of all incident injuries; 5 to 10% were fatal injuries; and the remaining injuries were either moderate or severe head injuries. The most complete tabulation of the outcome from acute brain injury comes from San Diego County in 1981 [11]. About 6% of the 2,972 admissions for brain injury died while in the hospital, and according to the Glasgow Outcome Scale, nearly 90% had a good recovery on discharge from the hospital. Almost 4% had moderate or severe outcomes, and 0.5% were discharged in a persistent vegetative state [11]. Between 5 and 10% of hospitalized brain-injured patients at discharge had apparent residual neurologic damage.

Based on the Olmsted County incidence rates reported for the years 1935 to 1974, incidence rates of head injury have increased progressively since 1945 [8]. In Olmsted County, since 1935 incidence more than doubled to its 1974 level of 200 head injuries per 100,000 population. Subsequent to World War II, most of the increase was due to increased numbers of mild injuries to both sexes, with little change in the incidence of moderate, severe, or fatal head injuries. The increased incidence occurred almost entirely within the ages of 15 to 24 for both sexes and was most pronounced during 1960 to 1970. The trend in mild injuries was associated with increasing numbers of motor vehicle accidents in this age interval and, to a lesser extent, was also associated with increased numbers of recreational injuries and assaults. The evident increase in mild injuries likely reflected a real increase in incidence and not an artifact of case ascertainment or changing utilization patterns of medical care [8].

The incidence data reported by the selected studies are approximate guides to the incidence of head and brain injury in the United States. The lack of standardized definitions and the inherent difficulties in identifying and classifying cases contribute to the uncertainty of any generalizations. However, the uncertainty does not appear to be extraordinary. Employing the general

Table 1.6 Percent Distribution of the External Causes of Head Injury as Reported in Selected Studies

Population and Year	Source	External Cause			
		Transportation	*Falls*	*Gunshot*	*Assault*
United States (1974)[a]	[19]	49%	28%	Not reported	
Olmsted County, Minn. (1965–1974)	[8]	47	29	3%	4%
San Diego County, Calif. (1978)	[9]	53	30	Not reported	11
North Central Virginia (1978)[a]	[18]	55	20	11	
Inner City Chicago, Ill. (1979)	[12]	31	20	6	34
Evanston, Ill. (1979)	[12]	37	27	1	15
Bronx County, N.Y. (1980)	[13]	31	29	33	
San Diego County, Calif. (1981)	[11]	48	21	6	12

[a]Excludes nonhospital deaths.

criteria of loss of consciousness, posttraumatic amnesia, confirmed intracranial injury, and skull fracture to define a case of head injury, the studies of large populations show incidence in the approximate range of 200 to 300 head injuries per 100,000 population per year. Based on these data, about 500,000 new cases of head or brain injury can be expected annually in the United States. Most, up to 70%, would be expected to be mild injuries. From 5 to 10% would be fatal injuries, the majority of which would be nonhospital deaths. From 5 to 10% of nonfatal injuries would be severe injuries, and the remaining would be moderate injuries. Of all cases discharged alive, up to 10% may have significant neurologic sequelae, with somewhat less than 1% discharged in a persistent vegetative state.

Male head injury incidence rates are twice female incidence rates, and male head injury mortality is three to four times greater than female mortality, a sex difference associated with pronounced male exposure to motor vehicle accidents and intentional injuries. The leading causes of head injury for both sexes are transportation accidents, falls, and violence. Transportation accidents can account for up to 50% of all head injuries, except in large, crowded, and deteriorating urban areas where interpersonal violence becomes a significant cause of head injury. Head injury particularly affects young adults and the elderly. The data are convincing: head injuries pose a significant and unique health problem in the United States.

RISK FACTORS AND PREVENTION

Individual risk factors for head injury have not been studied extensively in U.S. populations. Annegers et al [8] reported that after an initial head injury, the relative risk of a second head injury is tripled and that after a second injury, it increased to eight times that of the general population. The relative risk for second and subsequent head injuries was most pronounced among adults. The authors hypothesized that the greater increase of risk in adults was likely due to behavioral characteristics such as alcohol use. Alcohol use shortly before injury is the most common predisposing factor reported in head injury [5]. Psychological factors such as divorce and family disruption, socioeconomic factors, and preexisting psychiatric disorders have been cited in the literature as possible risk factors, but these findings have been debated [5].

What are the prospects for the prevention of head injuries or, more broadly, the prevention of intentional or unintentional injuries? Since there are no theoretical distinctions between injuries and disease [20], the prospects are at least as good, if not possibly better, than those that foreshadowed the decline and diminution of infectious disease. However, to realize significant gains we will have to adopt an epidemiologic approach to injuries that can illuminate the most sensitive and effective points for intervention. The models proposed by Haddon [20] that parallel models successfully used for the control of infectious disease serve that purpose.

The general epidemiologic model of injuries, proposed by Haddon, is based on the triad of host, agent, and environment. The host, the person at risk to injury, interacts with the agent of injury, physical energy, and with the environment of injury, the impacted structure. The interaction and physical energy interchange among the elements of the triad determine the timing, pathology, and severity of the injury [20]. From this view, each element of the triad presents itself as a potential point for intervention to disrupt the chain of events that leads to injury. The model applies to all phases of an injury and pinpoints interventions for the avoidance of injury and interventions to minimize the severity and sequelae of injury [21]. The goal of the epidemiologic model is to rank order interventions by their potential to achieve significant reductions in the frequency or severity of injury. Stated somewhat differently, the model recognizes not only individuals and their roles in the occurrence of injuries but also countermeasures directed at the environment to dissipate or eliminate the injurious nature of the physical energy interchange.

Successful applications of the Haddon model to a wide variety of injuries have been well reported [21]. These applications include the Flammable Fabrics Act, which dramatically reduced burns to children from flammable sleepwear; the Poison Prevention Act, which reduced fourfold the death rate of children less than 5 years old from poisonings due to regulated substances; the installation of window guards in New York City apartment houses, which significantly reduced deaths from falls; modifications of design features of motor vehicles that significantly reduced the frequency and severity of injuries in motor vehicle crashes; and modifications of highway designs that totally eliminated certain types of automobile crashes [21,22]. These are but a few of the examples of effective prevention strategies [21–24]. The extraordinary potential of motor vehicle occupant restraint systems to reduce head injuries and deaths is well established [23].

The most successful injury prevention strategies share an important feature. They provide automatic protection to the individual and do not rely on significant modifications of human behavior. They are based on the careful scientific observation that what was once thought to be human failure as a primary cause of injury is often actually human failure as the result of an unmanageable interaction with the vector or environment of injury or a secondary response to subtle environmental causes of injury [24]. Individuals do play a role in the incidence of injury, and individual culpability cannot be ignored, but major reductions in the incidence of injury are attainable with current technology that is automatic. Motor vehicle crashes, as we have seen, account for about half of all fatal and nonfatal head injuries. Robertson has argued that an effort to make cars more crashworthy could result in a 75% or greater reduction in highway fatalities in a decade [25]. Such an advance would reduce the incidence of head injury by at least one-half.

Are such estimates overoptimistic? Likely not if we consider that the United Kingdom has a death rate due to head injuries that is half the rate of the United States—a difference that can be attributed to prevention [15].

Similar arguments apply also to intentional injuries [22]. However, if prevention is ignored or resisted, then as Jennett wryly observed, there is no danger that a trauma surgeon will be out of work [15]. Conversely, success in injury prevention will prove to be another measure of the advancement of our civilization and the art, science, and practice of medicine and public health.

ACKNOWLEDGMENTS

This research was supported in part by the National Institutes of Health–National Institute of Neurological, Communicative Disorders, and Stroke, Contract NO1-NS-9-2314B.

REFERENCES

1. National Center for Health Statistics. Advance report, final mortality statistics, 1980. Monthly vital statistics report, vol. 32, no. 4, Suppl. DDHS pub. no. (PHS) 83–1120. Hyattsville, Md.: Public Health Service, August 1983.
2. Perloff JD, LeBailly SA, Kletke PR, Budette PP, Connelly JP. Premature death in the United States: years of life lost and health priorities. J Publ Health Policy 1984;5(2):167–84.
3. National Center for Health Statistics. Current estimates from the national health interview survey: United States, 1980. Series 10, no. 139. DDHS pub. no. (PHS) 82–1567. Hyattsville, Md.: Public Health Service, December 1981.
4. National Center for Health Statistics. Inpatient utilization of short-stay hospitals by diagnosis: United States, 1980. Series 13, no. 74. DDHS pub. no. (PHS) 83–1735. Hyattsville, Md.: Public Health Service, September 1983.
5. Levin HS, Benton AL, Grossman RG. Neurobehavioral consequences of closed head injury. New York: Oxford University Press, 1982.
6. Commission on Professional and Hospital Activities. The international classification of diseases, 9th revision. Clinical modification. Ann Arbor: Edwards Brothers, Inc., 1978.
7. National Center for Health Statistics. Multiple causes of death in the United States. Monthly vital statistics report, vol. 32, no. 10, Suppl. 2. DDHS pub. no. (PHS) 84–1120. Hyattsville, Md.: Public Health Service, February 17, 1984.
8. Annegers JF, Grabow JD, Kurland LT. The incidence, causes, and secular trends of head trauma in Olmsted County, Minnesota. Neurology 1980;30:912–19.
9. Klauber MR, Barrett-Connor E, Marshall LF. The epidemiology of head injury: a prospective study of an entire community—San Diego County, California, 1978. Am J. Epidemiol 113:500–09.
10. Frankowski RF, Klauber MR, Tabaddor K. Head injury mortality: a comparison of three metropolitan counties. NINCDS report (manuscript).
11. Kraus JF, Black MA, Hessol N. The incidence of acute brain injury and serious impairment in a defined population. Am J Epidemiol 1984;119:186–201.
12. Whitman S, Coonley-Hoganson R, Desai BT. Comparative head trauma experi-

ences in two socioeconomically different Chicago-area communities: a population study. Am J Epidemiol 1984;119:186–201.
13. Cooper KD, Tabaddor K, Hauser WA. The epidemiology of head injury in the Bronx. Neuroepidemiology 1983;2:70–88.
14. Spain DM, Fox RI, Marcus A. Evaluation of hospital care in one trauma care system. Am J Public Health 1984;74:1122–25.
15. Jennett B, Teasdale G. Management of head injuries. Philadelphia: F.A. Davis Company, 1981.
16. Jennett B, MacMillian R. Epidemiology of head injuries. Br Med J 1981;282:101–04.
17. Frankowski RF, Annegers JF, Whitman S. The descriptive epidemiology of head trauma in the United States. In: Becker DP, Povlishock JT, eds. Central Nervous System Research Status Report, 1985. Bethesda, Md.: NINCDS, 1985;33–43.
18. Jagger J, Levine JI, Jane JA. Epidemiologic features of head injury in a predominantly rural population. J Trauma 1984;24:40–44.
19. Anderson DW, McLaurin RL. Report on the national head and spinal cord injury survey. J Neurosurg (suppl.) 1980;53:S1–S43.
20. Haddon W, Jr. Advances in the epidemiology of injuries as a basis for public policy. Publ Health Rep 1980;95:411–21.
21. Robertson LS. Injuries; causes, control strategies and public policy. Lexington, Mass.: D.C. Heath and Company, Lexington Books, 1983.
22. Baker SP, O'Neill B, Karpf RS. The injury fact book. Lexington, Mass.: D.C. Heath and Company, Lexington Books, 1984.
23. Office of Technology Assessment. Background paper #1: mandatory passive restraint systems in automobiles: issues and evidence. Technology and handicapped people. Pub. no. OTA-BP-H-15. Congress of the United States, Washington, D.C.: OTA, September 1982.
24. Waller JA. Injury control: a guide to the causes and prevention of trauma. Lexington, Mass.: D.C. Heath and Company, Lexington Books, 1985.
25. Robertson LS. Highway injury. Texas Med 1983;79:48–50.

Chapter 2

Ensuring against Tragedy: The Decision to Treat the Severely Head Injured

H. Tristram Engelhardt, Jr.

Modern medical technology raises a number of difficult moral issues. Not the least of these is the question of when to employ that technology if the costs are high, the chance of success is unclear, and the quality of outcome is likely to be less than full health. Such issues are especially salient in the case of head injuries. They are complicated by the fact that it is often difficult initially to judge with certainty the likelihood and quality of success. Still, where general solutions are not available, partial solutions have merit. To avoid the boonless commitment of resources, there is the need to develop more precise and reliable indications of when therapeutic interventions will not be successful. One might think here of the use of the trauma score [1] as a predictor of likelihood of survival [2] or of the development of other indicators of survival [3].

The investment of significant resources in treatment unlikely to be of benefit raises serious moral questions. The more one invests in health care, the less one can invest in other important human undertakings. Moreover, major investments in health care require major redistributions of resources— a problem that raises questions regarding the proper limits of state authority. In addition, the ability to set limits to investments in health care is integral to our being in command of technology rather than technology's controlling us.

A TRADITION OF RESTRAINT

As Amundsen has shown, the commitment to saving life at all costs is one without classical roots [4]. The usual and customary standards of care in the ancient world committed the physician to not treating hopeless cases.* The

---

*The author of The Hippocratic Treatise *The Art* enjoins physicians to "refuse to treat those who are overmastered by their diseases, realizing that in such cases medicine is powerless." The art, vol. III. In: Jones WHS, trans. Hippocrates. Cambridge: Harvard University Press, 1959;193.

grounds for physicians' reticence to treat in such circumstances were complex. It in part stemmed from a concern not to bring medicine into disregard through glaring failures. This approach reflected as well the Greco-Roman moral commitment to moderation. An element of the human condition as that of a finite being was to accept the inevitability of death and not to struggle vainly to hold to life when such a struggle only prolongs death.* These views were developed in a context where hubris was to be avoided and where technological promises were not present to tempt to hubris.

These same issues were addressed within the context of the Christian West. Christians came to hold that it was an obligation of physicians to treat patients, even when patients did not have funds to purchase care [5]. There were always limits to such obligations, however [6]. With the Renaissance and increasing expectations from medicine, the question of limits was explored in detail [7]. Questions were raised in the context of a nun, priest, or monk seeking to determine when he or she was not obliged to accept treatment requested by a religious superior [8]. These questions were generalized to the laity as well. The response was that one was not obliged to provide treatment if it would not be useful (*nemo ad inutile tenetur*). Moreover, one was not required to submit to treatment if it would only postpone the inevitable (*parum pro nihilo reputatur mortaliter*) [9].

These discussions framed the classic distinctions between ordinary and extraordinary care where ordinary care was obligatory care and extraordinary care was that that constituted an undue inconvenience and therefore could not be imposed on a patient. In generating this distinction, theologians took into account not just costs but also pain and even revulsion toward a particular treatment (*horror magnus*). This approach continued to be applied and received an influential modern rearticulation when Pius XII discussed the question of providing treatment for individuals with serious brain damage in a statement issued November 24, 1957 [10]. His statements were written against the background of the development of intensive care units during the 1950s.

One should note the extent to which the pope adapted his moral considerations to the financial and psychological resources of the individual, the family, and society.

> Normally one is held to use only ordinary means—according to circumstances of persons, places, times, and culture—that is to say, means that do not involve any grave burden for oneself or another. A more strict obligation would be too burdensome for most men and would render the attainment of the higher, more important good too difficult (pp. 395–96). [10]

This approach by the pope is integral to a conservative religious viewpoint. If one believes in an afterlife, there can be a disproportion in investing all the

---

*Seneca, for example, states that "Life is not to be bought at all costs." Letter 70. In: Hadas M, trans. The stoic philosophy of Seneca. New York: W.W. Norton, 1958:203.

resources at one's disposal in prolonging life. As Pius XII expressed it, "Life, health, all temporal activities are in fact subordinated to spiritual ends" (p. 396) [10]. An unrestrained investment in life-prolonging interventions is more plausible against the modern view that "you only go around once."

A SOCIETY'S INSURANCE AGAINST CATASTROPHES

In the absence of the religious beliefs like those of the pope, there remain substantial secular reasons for investing less than all disposable resources in saving lives [11]. Even if this is the only life one is likely to have, one must still decide how to husband resources to maximize its quality. If one commits all resources to prolonging life, none will be left for enjoying the life one seeks to prolong. One must strike a balance. One cannot protect against all catastrophes. The development of health care systems, intensive care units, and indications for treatment reflect the final common pathway of various decisions between investing funds in prolonging life versus the fleeting pleasures of this transient existence. The difficulty is that these issues have not been clearly and explicitly addressed in public policy debates.

The problem of making such allocational choices is faced by societies as they establish social programs to blunt the outcomes of the natural and social lotteries. All individuals are exposed to the vicissitudes of the natural lottery, the outcomes of natural forces that lead some to early deaths and others to long and healthy lives, as well as the social lottery, the outcomes of individual and societal actions and choices and also to some having the resources for the purchase of health care while others are left medically indigent.* By providing a particular level of care against a certain range of risks, a society takes out what is equivalent to an insurance policy against the adverse outcomes of the natural and social lotteries. Such insurance must be envisaged as being established before the adverse occurrence. One cannot take out extra flood insurance as the waters rise in one's home. The decision about the amount of funds one wishes to invest in flood insurance versus the amount to be devoted to health insurance, housing, entertainment, etc. must be understood as being made before any risks of the flood are realized. Rationality requires planning before catastrophes.

Since costly preparation for possible catastrophes competes with other allocations of funds, one needs a means for assessing the relative appropriateness of particular investments in particular forms of insurance against the untoward outcomes of the natural and social lotteries. Such choices require assigning a value to human life in the sense of deciding among competing

---

*I use the terms "natural lottery" and "social lottery" not to identify the distributions of natural and social assets, but rather to identify the forces that effect the distribution.

investments. For instance, if one routinely provides $30,000 worth of treatment for individuals who have suffered head injuries and have only one chance in a hundred of surviving, then one has assigned a value of $3 million to such individuals' lives. The public policy question is the extent to which we wish to embrace policies that involve such levels of expenditure with such a low level of return. The decision will depend in part on how often such choices have to be made. If one rarely commits $100,000 to saving the life of an individual when there is only 1% chance of success, one may decide that a $10 million valuation of life under such circumstances can be tolerated as an exception. Such a policy ceases to be prudent the more frequently such decisions are made. Unchecked, the policy would lead to substantial transfers from the enterprises that make life worth living (art museums, operas, parks, and sports events) to the prolongation and saving of life. In short, one seeks a balance between investing resources in enjoying life versus prolonging life.

Such choices admittedly are painful. In making them, one acknowledges that one is a mere mortal and abandons the fantasy that human life can or should be saved at any cost. Again, such an acknowledgment appears to be more easily made within the context of religions that sustain an expectation of an afterlife. One theologian argued that (in 1940s dollars) one was not obliged to invest more than $2,000 in saving a life, no matter how rich an individual might be [12]. In any event, it has been traditionally acknowledged that burdens defeat obligations of beneficence. One is obliged to come to the aid of others only when that endeavor does not constitute a severe burden. As already noted, the less likely the success, the more the duty was acknowledged to be weakened. In fact, there are passages in traditional Christian reflections on these matters to suggest that quality of life considerations may play a role as well in that the obligation to treat is weakened as the probability of restoring an individual to full health diminishes.

It is also worthwhile noting that traditional approaches to obligations to treat allow for discrimination on the basis of the quality of life. Once one has established the basic duty of beneficence with regard to the treatment of injured individuals, one can always decide to be supererogatory in a discriminatory fashion. One may decide to do more, to assume more financial and psychological burdens than are minimally required. But one need not. Where only courageous (i.e., more than morally required) labors can restore an individual to full health, one may decide to forgo treatment when the life secured will likely be marked by severe mental and physical handicaps.

In the secular terms of a social insurance policy, these matters can be put fairly straightforwardly with respect to the circumstances under which one would wish to set resources aside to provide for treatment. The less likely the success and the more limited the quality of success, the less reasonable it is for individuals or society to invest in interventions to preserve life. Given the insurance metaphor, the question is the extent to which individuals would purchase coverage (or invest funds in establishing systems to care) for treatment for themselves, should they sustain head injuries where there is likely to be a poor quality of life.

In this context, this question is not equivalent to the question of whether one would choose to die under such circumstances of poor quality of life; it is the question of whether one would invest resources to be able to live under such circumstances. One may indeed accept life of a diminished quality once the resources have been expended in securing it. However, it is another question entirely whether one will set aside resources to be used in the event that they are needed to save life, if that life is to be marked by substantial mental and physical handicaps. The poorer the likely quality of life, the less likely it is that rational persons would choose to invest funds in such insurance against the loss of the natural and social lotteries. Though one might decide to set funds aside for treatment of oneself (and others), in the case where $30,000 of investment would secure a one-out-of-a-hundred chance of recovery of an acceptable level of health, one might not choose such an investment if nine times out of ten one's survival would be marred by considerable intellectual deficits and physical handicaps. In such circumstances, the purchase price for a full return to health would presume a value of $30 million since there would be a one-out-of-a-thousand chance of return to an acceptable level of health. In short, a reasonable moral basis can be secured for a public policy that would not support the investment of significant funds in the treatment of individuals likely to survive with poor quality of life.

In addition, it is likely that reasonable men and women will take into consideration the length of life likely to be secured by any costly health care intervention. One may decide, for example, not to set aside funds that would restore one to full functional capacities following a head injury in circumstances when one is suffering from a concurrent rapidly terminal disease. The less life to be secured, the less worthwhile it becomes to set aside funds for preservation of life under such circumstances. One can express the relationship between the obligation of beneficence and the costs involved, the probability of success, the likely quality of life, and the probable length of survival in the following fashion:

$$\frac{\text{Obligation}}{\text{of beneficence}} = \frac{\text{Probability of success} \times \text{Quality of life} \times \text{Length of life}}{\text{Costs}}$$

As the equation indicates, with an increase in costs the obligation of beneficence is weakened. As I have suggested, costs should be interpreted broadly, as has traditionally been the case, to include not only economic costs but also social and psychological costs (e.g., a *horror magnus,* or a great revulsion to the treatment). Further, as the likelihood, quality, and quantity of the success diminish, so does the obligation of beneficence weaken.

It is unlikely that we will find convincing mechanisms simply to discover the exact point at which the obligation of beneficence is defeated (e.g., $2,000 1940s dollars). The insurance metaphor underscores the fact that men and women must create an understanding of the point at which the obligation of beneficence is defeated through their decisions to purchase or not to purchase insurance against particular untoward events. As a culture armed with expensive medical technologies, we have the burden of deciding the extent to which we wish to establish societal insurance programs that will pay for medical interventions when the costs are considerable and the likelihood of benefit limited.

We are returned to the need to assemble better data regarding the likelihood and quality of success, given different levels of injury so as to create prudent public policy. This research will commit society and the medical professions to the further elaboration of indications for treatment and continued treatment. Classically, indications for treatment have balanced likely benefits with possible morbidity and mortality due to the treatment [13]. The suggestion here is that considerations of cost should be incorporated as well. This is, in fact, not a radical suggestion. Most talk about unnecessary hysterectomies or other surgical procedures does not simply focus on an improper balance of benefits and risks to the patient but also incorporates the notion that the benefits likely to be secured may not be worth the cost. Recent discussions about eliminating routine chest X-rays on admission to hospitals [14] or routine urinalysis [15] do not simply allege that the X-rays or urinalyses are likely to cause more harm than benefit to the patient involved but that their costs are not justified by the likely returns (in the case of urinalysis, a modification is suggested rather than a complete abolishment of the practice).

Better data regarding the likely outcome of interventions, given different levels of trauma, will allow informed public debate and the fashioning of prudent policy regarding the use of expensive medical interventions. Such data are part of writing the fine print of a basic social insurance policy for a high technology culture. Given the character of emergency interventions, such public policy will need to acknowledge the fact that it will often make sense to treat aggressively and then to reassess the commitment to treatment as more complete data are acquired: an initial commitment to treatment is not a commitment to continue treatment, irrespective of new and more complete data that indicate that further intervention is no longer warranted. Often, without a clear moral argument, it is assumed that simply because one has initiated treatment or intubated a patient, one may not cease treatment, in that failing to treat is simply an inaction, while extubating a patient or turning off a respirator is an action. But there is as much of an action involved in continuing to power a respirator as is involved in the initial intubation and activation of the respirator. In short, previous treatment does not of itself morally commit one to continue treatment once it is clear that the established indications for treatment are no longer satisfied than it obliges one to initiate treatment under such circumstances. This becomes clearer through use of the insurance metaphor because reassessment and discontinuation of treatment can express the consequences of commitments made in advance of injury.

Though the analysis in this chapter has often focused on individual decisions, the intention has been to invoke the model of individuals joined together in fashioning general societal policies. This is, in fact, the mechanism through which democracies dispose of their commonly owned resources. A full account of the moral issues involved in the recruitment of such resources cannot be given here [16]. Here it is enough to indicate that responsible use of technology will require securing not only data regarding its costs but also indications on the basis of which fairly reliable predictions can be made with regard to the likelihood and quality of success. Individuals and societies will need to recognize that the worlds of science and technology are worlds of probability and that judicious choices require decisions made not on the basis of certainties but reasonable likelihoods of outcome.

THE COUNSELS OF FINITUDE

Both religious and secular approaches lead individuals and societies to recognize the conditions of human finitude. Humans never have infinite resources and rarely certain data on the basis of which to make decisions, even those decisions most important for their lives. As a result, individual choices and public policy must be framed on the basis of limited resources and likely outcomes. Those who expect an afterlife can understand such choices in terms of seeing a policy of saving lives at any cost as an idolatry of this physical life to the detriment of more important undertakings. Within the context of secular reflections, one must acknowledge that, if one purchases life at any cost, there will not be sufficient resources to make the lives saved by such policies worth living. The human condition is one of limitation and compromise.

Though one may have sympathies with the general high moral tone of laments about the negative effects of economic considerations on the emergency care given to individuals with severe head and other injuries [17], one must still recognize that there will be no simple answers and that the provision of care under all circumstances is one of the simple answers to be avoided. In addition, the more one pursues cost constraints, the more one in fact limits funds for cost shifting and, thereby, indirectly sets policy with regard to indications for treatment when the costs are high and the outcomes uncertain. In an editorial, Relman states, "Surely economic considerations should be subordinated to the patient's interest" [18]. Indeed, discussions of these issues often proceed as if medical justifications for treatment or transfer should be made independent of economic and other considerations. This chapter suggests a rephrasing of Relman's point. Economic considerations must play a role in fashioning such judgments, though surely not the only role. Economic considerations are always part of the choices made in the face of uncertainty by finite beings with limited resources. This is a conclusion in morality that, with qualifications, should be acceptable from both religious and secular points of view.

REFERENCES

1. Champion HR, Sacco WJ, Carnazzo AJ. Trauma score. Crit Care Med 1981;9:672–76.
2. Champion HR. Reported in National Center for Health Services Research Grant No. R18HS02559.
3. Knaus WA, Zimmerman JE, Wagner DF. APACHE—acute physiology and chronic health evaluation: a physiologically based classification system. Crit Care Med 1981;9:591–97; Knaus WA, Draper EA, Wagner DP. Toward quality review in intensive care: the APACHE system. QRB 1983; 196–204; Knaus WA, Draper EA, Wagner DP. The use of intensive care: new research initiatives and their implications for national health policy. Milbank Memorial Fund Quar 1983;61:561–83.
4. Amundsen D. The physician's obligation to prolong life: a medical duty without classical roots. Hastings Ctr 1978;8:23–80.
5. Amundsen D. Casuistry and professional obligations: the regulation of physicians by the court of conscience in the late middle ages, Part II. Transactions and Studies of the Coll of Physicians of Phil 1981;3:93–95.
6. Aquinas T. Summa theologica II-II, 71, 1.
7. Janini J. La operation quirurgica, remedio ordinario. Revista Espanola de Teologia 1958;18:331–48.
8. McCartney JJ. The development of the doctrine of ordinary and extraordinary means of preserving life in Catholic moral theology before the Karen Quinlan case. Linacre Quar 1980;47:215–24.
9. Kelly G. The duty of using artificial means of preserving life. Theological Studies 1950;11:203–20.
10. Pius XII. The prolongation of life. The Pope Speaks 1958;4:393–98.
11. Engelhardt HT, Jr. Shattuck lecture—allocation of scarce medical resources and the availability of organ transplantation. NEJM 1984;311:66–71.
12. Healy EF. Cited in: Kelly G. The duty of using artificial means of preserving life. Theological Studies 1950;11:206.
13. Nordenfelt L, Lindahl BIB, eds. Health, disease, and causal explanations in medicine. Dordrecht, Holland: Reidel, 1984.
14. Hubbell FA. The impact of routine admission chest X-ray films on patient care. NEJM 1985;312:209–13.
15. Shaw ST, Poon SY, Wong ET. Routine urinalysis: is the dipstick enough? AMA 1985;253:1596–1600.
16. Engelhardt HT, Jr. The foundations of bioethics. New York: Oxford, 1985.
17. Wrenn K. Sounding board: no insurance, no admission. NEJM 1985;312:373–74.
18. Relman AS. Economic considerations in emergency care. NEJM 1985;312:372–73.

Part I

Acute Treatment of Head Injured Patients

Michael E. Miner
Dennis R. Kopaniky

Since the landmark paper of Cushing's experience in World War I, neurosurgeons have been studying how to better the acute treatment of head injured patients [1]. Even in that experience of 70 years ago, early aggressive treatment was advocated because the results, in terms of salvaged lives, improved. Laboratory investigation had previously made it clear that brain injury resulted in multiple systemic effects that might, in turn, affect the injured brain [2]. Thus, the study of brain injury and its complex effects on other organ systems can be traced nearly to the inception of modern neurosurgery. Since the 1960s we have witnessed more sophisticated instrumentation with which to monitor more brain-related functions, as well as the development of a productive relationship between neurosurgeons, anesthesiologists, and neurologists, all interested in the acutely brain-injured patient. We have come to recognize the importance not only of the systemic effects of brain injury but also the remote effects. The six chapters in this part continue the tradition of the holistic approach to the patient with brain injury.

The acute life-sustaining organs are the brain, heart, and lungs. That diminished function of the heart or lungs affects brain metabolism is a basic tenet of cardiopulmonary resuscitation. Chapter 3 points out that it is a two-way street because brain injury may also severely affect heart and lung function, and the interplay between these organ systems is vital to patient survival. Hand in glove with this is the recognition of the importance of monitoring and treating increased intracranial pressure. Chapter 4 describes regimens for treating increased intracranial pressure that require an understanding of cardiopulmonary function. It also observes that most of the treatments used to lower intracranial pressure affect cardiopulmonary function. Indeed, some of these regimens may lower intracranial pressure by virtue of their cardiopulmonary effects.

Investigations into the complex problems of brain injury are becoming increasingly based on physiological data derived at the bedside. The study of brain and systemic metabolism is fundamental to understanding brain injury. Chapter 5 describes a sophisticated bedside technique of continuously monitoring cerebral oxygen extraction and how those data can be used to fine tune acute treatment. Compelling arguments are presented that this may become an important treatment tool. Systemic metabolism, nutrition, is just beginning to be appreciated as being altered by head injury and, in turn, altering the outcome of brain injury. Chapter 6 evaluates the literature and contributes new understanding to this complex problem. Although we commonly accept nutrition as one of life's basic needs, the metabolic needs after brain injury are not well studied and not well met.

Consortium studies allow observations to be cross checked between centers and low incidence phenomena to be evaluated. The report from the National Traumatic Coma Bank in Chapter 6 details both the independence and interrelations between clinically relevant variables in predicting the quality of recovery after head injury. Chapter 8 describes the advances made in predicting what lesions more commonly result in posttraumatic epilepsy. In addition, the chapter reviews the science that supports the current standards of practice in prophylactically treating these patients for seizures. It points out that the study of posttraumatic epilepsy needs to continue, in search of both better medications and better treatment regimens.

The treatment of brain-injured patients requires a holistic approach from its very inception—holistic in terms of integrating the effects of treatment on the entire organism and in terms of distant effects like the delayed onset of posttraumatic seizures. The fundamental basis of the acute treatment of brain injury is to provide the physiologic milieu for the brain to heal and to prevent untoward secondary effects from the injury. The chapters in this part continue the tradition of dissecting the complex effects of brain injury, studying the parts, and integrating treatment so that the rehabilitative phase of recovery can yield the highest quality of survival.

REFERENCES

1. Cushing H. Concerning operations for the craniocerebral wounds of modern warfare. Milit Surg 1916;38:601–15.
2. Cushing H. Concerning a definite regulatory mechanism of the vasomotor centre which controls blood pressure during cerebral compression. Johns Hopkins Hosp Bull 1901;12:290.

Chapter 3

Cardiopulmonary Changes after Head Injury

Elizabeth A.M. Frost
Michael F. Domurat

Examination of the pulse was used as a prognostic indicator of head injury 4,000 years ago in China [1]. Over 200 years ago a Scottish anatomist, John Hunter, correlated altered states of consciousness and variations in respiratory patterns [2]. However, not until relatively recently, in 1897, did Horsley and Kramer observe that death after head injury was usually due to respiratory arrest [3]. They postulated that if respiration could be supported, the brain might survive. In a classic paper in 1901, Walter B. Cannon described the prototype of the Richmond bolt. He monitored intracranial pressure (ICP), noted the effects of respiration, and concluded that support of the respiratory system would improve survival [4].

Recent improvement in survival rates after major intracranial injury can be attributed to improvement in ancillary systems rather than to advances in surgical techniques. Such improvements include better cardiopulmonary support, more accurate diagnosis, faster transportation to tertiary care facilities, and better education of paramedical personnel.

RESPIRATORY PROBLEMS ASSOCIATED WITH HEAD TRAUMA

A review of 116 patients who talked after head injury but subsequently died (a situation reported to occur in 38% of cases) revealed that one or more avoidable complications occurred in 70% of cases. In 54%, these complications contributed directly to death [5]. The most commonly listed abnormalities were hypoxia, hypotension, delay in treatment, sepsis, and seizures. Iatrogenic factors such as misplacement of endotracheal tubes, pneumothorax following subclavian puncture, hematomas in the neck after angiography, and fractured ribs caused by overzealous resuscitation are complications known to us all but rarely published (perhaps for medicolegal reasons).

Hypoxia is by far the most common preventable event following head injury. Establishment and maintenance of the so-called impeccable airway is of paramount importance.

We undertook a study to differentiate between central and peripheral causes of respiratory dysfunction, to assess the effect of early hypoxemia on outcome and to determine the value of intensive respiratory care for pulmonary dysfunction [6]. Causes of respiratory insufficiency in a group of 100 patients are outlined in Figure 3.1. In 70% of patients, mostly young, otherwise healthy, males, we were unable to find any cause of the hypoxia other than the head injury. Central neurogenic hyperventilation was a pattern that occurred frequently. Minute ventilation may increase to as much as 40 l. Hypoxia was caused by the intense work of breathing and the shift of the O_2 dissociation curve to the left due to respiratory alkalosis.

In our study, four patients developed pulmonary edema. In two instances this was probably related to osmotic diuretic therapy to control ICP hypertension. The first case, a newborn, developed pulmonary edema shortly after infusion of 1 gm mannitol. In the second instance, a 70-year-old man with a history of hypertension and heart disease became cyanotic after receiving 10 gm mannitol over a 15 min period. Experience suggests that in both these cases, furosemide 1 mg/kg would have been a better choice. In the other two cases, which were less clearly defined, we would suggest that neurogenic pulmonary edema was a factor that increased hypoxia although this syndrome has been a point of controversy [7,8]. It has been demonstrated in experimental head trauma that probably resulted from a centrally mediated massive sympathetic discharge perhaps secondary to hypothalamic impairment [9–11]. Shift of blood from the high resistance systemic circulation to the low resistance pulmonary circulation causes an increase in pulmonary vascular pressure and blood volume, which increases hydrostatic pressure with hemorrhage and edema. Surfactant becomes inactivated and atelectasis and hypoxia develop.

Disseminated intravascular coagulopathy and fibrinolysis syndrome were documented in two patients although abnormalities of clotting parameters can

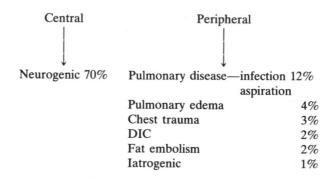

Figure 3.1 Causes of respiratory insufficiency after head injury.

be identified in the majority of patients after major head injury [12]. The brain is a very rich source of tissue thromboplastin that may be released after cranial injury, causing both hemorrhage and thrombotic events [13]. Treatment requires prompt administration of fresh frozen plasma, cryoprecipitate, and platelets [14].

Fat embolism was the cause of hypoxia in 2% of cases, both associated with long bone fractures. Although occurrence of fat embolism after such fractures has been estimated at between 10 and 25%, in large autopsy studies, 80 to 100% of patients who die of various causes after fractures of long bones have fat emboli in their lungs [15]. Disruption of the surface negative charge in chylomicrons after trauma causes coalescence that can occlude small vessels. Clinical diagnosis is made by the presence of tachycardia, hypoxia, electrocardiographic changes, and embolic phenomena evidenced in the nail beds, retinae, sclerae, and skin. Treatment requires cardiac and respiratory support, infusion of aminophylline, narcotics, steroids, and low molecular weight dextran. Use of alcohol and heparin is controversial.

The second part of our study assessed the effect of hypoxemia on outcome. We found that the initial calculated pulmonary shunt in patients with a good outcome was 8.9% (± 5.5). In patients who survived but with deficit, the shunt was 13.6% (± 4.5) and in those who died, 15.6% (± 6.1). Only 24% of patients in the improved group had an initial shunt over 10%, while 54% of patients in the group surviving with deficit and 80% of those who died exhibited this degree of hypoxemia.

We concluded that initial pulmonary shunt was a prognostic indicator in head injury. However, of more importance is that all patients must be considered hypoxic until proven otherwise. The cause of respiratory dysfunction is due to intracranial damage in 70% of cases. Since blood samples collected within minutes of injury showed decreased oxygen saturation, we felt that hypoxia can develop almost immediately after injury.

Diagnosis of Respiratory Insufficiency

A patient requires respiratory support if the respiratory pattern is irregular, if the rate rises above 40/min or falls below 10/min, if the tidal volume is less than 1.5 cc/kg and the vital capacity below 1 l. In the head-injured patient, development of hypercarbia ($PaCO_2 > 45$ mm Hg) or hypoxemia ($PaO_2 < 70$ mm Hg) also indicates the need for ventilatory support.

Although clinically specific abnormalities of respiratory rate pattern have been correlated with the level of the central nervous system lesion, such changes are more consistently related to extent and bilaterality [16,17]. In general, a eupneic pattern of breathing indicates a small, unilateral lesion, and outcome is good. The presence of Cheyne-Stokes respiration indicates a bilateral lesion. Mortality rates exceed 50%. Apneustic patterns may indicate pontine infarction but may also be caused by drug intoxication, hypoglycemia, or severe anemia.

Prognosis is, again, poor. Ataxic respiration usually results from a posterior fossa lesion with medullary compression. Outcome is usually fatal [18].

Therapy

The aim of therapy is to achieve PaO_2 levels above 100 mm Hg and $PaCO_2$ levels of 27 to 30 mm Hg. Frequently, adequate respiration may be achieved simply by tilting the head back, clearing the mouth, and inserting an airway. Supplemental oxygen should always be given. If these measures do not suffice, intubation should be performed and ventilation supported. Because of the high related incidence of narcotic overdose in head injury, naloxone hydrochloride is often indicated. The method of intubating the trachea is important as laryngoscopy and the passage of an endotracheal tube in a semiconscious, struggling youth may cause a 200 to 300% increase in ICP. Administration of succinylcholine and the attendant fasciculation do not increase ICP per se, but as $PaCO_2$ increases during apnea and insertion of the laryngoscope, ICP still rises. A bolus infusion of sodium thiopental (250 mg) decreases ICP in about 60 seconds and is therefore an appropriate drug choice prior to intubation. Although it is difficult to administer hypnotic agents to patients already comatose, this is an essential maneuver to avoid potentially disastrous increases in ICP. The sequence of events should be (1) application of cricoid pressure to diminish chances of aspiration; (2) ventilation with 100% O_2 and AMBU bag; (3) intravenous administration of sodium pentothal 3 mg/kg with or without lidocaine 1 mg/kg; (4) continued ventilation; (5) intubation. Any period of apnea will be accompanied by a rise in ICP even though the $PaCO_2$ may remain within a relatively hypocapnic range (e.g., 27 to 33 mm Hg over 1 min). Similarly, suctioning, if it is not preceded by hyperventilation and sodium pentothal injection, will increase ICP. Bucking due to inadequate respiratory control or insufficient sedation increases ICP and may initiate pressure waves.

Mechanical Ventilation

Although intubation secures the airway, assisted ventilation may still be necessary to ensure adequate tissue oxygenation and carbon dioxide removal. An early study showed a significant increase in good survivors and a decrease in mortality in patients treated with controlled hyperventilation [19].

Several terms have been applied to mechanical ventilatory patterns. Controlled ventilation (CV) is applicable to patients in whom there is no respiratory effort (severe brain stem injury, narcotic overdose). This ventilatory mode is also essential for patients paralyzed by muscle relaxants (used to achieve control in central neurogenic hyperventilation or to prevent bucking and increase in central venous pressure if ICP is high). Intermittent positive pressure breathing

(IPPB) was used both as prophylaxis and in prevention of pneumonic consolidation [20]. However, both application and removal of this mode may be associated with increases in ICP and initiation of plateau waves. Moreover, because hypoxia may develop after IPPB is withdrawn, it is no longer recommended [21].

Positive end expiratory pressure (PEEP) added to the expiratory limb increases functional residual capacity by increasing mean airway pressure, decreases the alveolar-arterial oxygen tension gradient (A-aDO_2), and increases PaO_2. It is usually then possible to reduce the inspired oxygen concentration and maintain an adequate PaO_2. Normally, 5 cm H_2O PEEP is applied initially and, if cardiac stability is maintained, may be increased. Early concerns of a deleterious effect of PEEP on intracranial dynamics are unfounded [22,23]. If the patient is nursed in a 30° head-up position, there is sufficient interposed venous system to prevent direct transmission of pressure from the chest to the head. As oxygenation improves, intracranial compliance increases and ICP usually reverts to more normal levels.

The current ventilatory modes of choice are continuous positive airway pressure (CPAP) in combination with intermittent mandatory ventilation (IMV). This latter technique was originally introduced in the sequence of weaning patients from ventilators but has been found to be a useful means of augmenting spontaneous ventilation rather than providing total support [24].

Jet ventilation, or high frequency positive pressure ventilation, was developed as an experimental method to abolish respiratory-induced fluctuations in blood pressure that interfered with measurement of carotid sinus reflex [25]. Several systems using rates that delivered 60 to 100 breaths/min were developed. Success in short operations like endoscopy was demonstrated. The emphasis of usefulness shifted to maintenance of cardiovascular stability from reduction of barotrauma [26].

Finally, high frequency oscillation (HFO) has been developed to control gas transport in the lungs [27]. Normally, gas transport is achieved by cyclic ventilation with bulk flow and diffuse movement within alveoli. When the force of the beating heart is transmitted to the surrounding lung tissue, diffuse transport of gases in the lung periphery speeds up some fivefold (the phenomenon of cardiogenic mixing) [28]. HFO uses a more energetic mix applied to the airway (300 or more oscillations/min). This ventilatory mode has been used successfully in the treatment of respiratory failure when conventional means of promoting gas transport and distribution have proved inadequate [29].

Advantages of high frequency ventilation include reduction of barotrauma, maintenance of cardiovascular stability, homogeneous gas mixing, reduction of peak airway pressure and ICP, inhibition of spontaneous respiratory drive, and decreased brain movement [30]. Adequate oxygenation (which may, however, be less than that achieved by standard volume ventilation) and elimination of carbon dioxide are maintained for hours or days. However, several complications have been described including development of problems related to lack of humidification and temperature maintenance, excessive pressure development with lung rupture, air trapping, hyperventilation, and carbon dioxide retention.

Preliminary studies have indicated that high frequency ventilation is particularly advantageous as an aid in the healing of acutely traumatized lungs (e.g., post aspiration, adult respiratory distress syndrome) [31].

CARDIAC CHANGES

Cushing described a combination of hypertension and bradycardia associated with raised ICP [32]. By the time this clinical picture is present, ICP unfortunately has reached diastolic blood pressure levels and the patient is usually brain dead. The importance of Cushing's observation was to focus attention on the cardiovascular system in the head-injured patient.

Vital Signs

Normovolemic hypotension following closed head injury is rare in the absence of major scalp lacerations and multiple trauma (usually splenic rupture). Brain stem injury and destruction of the vasomotor center in the medulla are incompatible with life [33]. Theoretically, hypotension could occur in hypertensive patients chronically receiving catecholamine-depleting antihypertensive medications.

The most frequently observed hemodynamic abnormalities are hypertension and tachycardia. Increases of mean arterial pressure as much as 29% and heart rate of 56% have been described [34]. The same authors found less consistent increases in pulmonary artery pressure, pulmonary capillary wedge pressure, and peripheral vascular resistance. In another study, tachycardia over 120 beats/min was reported in one-third of head-injured patients and systolic blood pressure of over 160 mm Hg in one-fourth on admission [35]. Examination of eighty-six patients in our emergency room shortly after injury showed similar results.

Electrocardiographic and Myocardial Changes

The most common electrocardiographic (EKG) abnormalities include prolongation of the QT_c interval and increased voltage of the P waves. QT_c interval prolongations over 0.54 sec (normal 0.24 to 0.44 sec) are common as are P wave voltages of 2.5 mm or more. Thirty-nine percent of P wave changes were associated with heart rates of 55 to 90, suggesting that they may be due not to elevated catecholamines levels but to direct stimulation of certain areas of the brain. Other EKG abnormalities include precordial ST segment elevations, U waves, inverted T waves, and bundle-branch block [36]. The number of abnormalities has been shown to increase in proportion to the severity of the trauma as measured by the Glasgow Coma Scale (GCS).

Some investigators have noted a correlation between outcome and QT_c prolongation, with an interval of 0.44 to 0.49 sec corresponding to a mortality rate double that of patients with normal QT_c intervals. A tripling of the mortality rate is associated with extremely prolonged QT_c intervals [14].

Characteristic EKG changes and myocardial lesions have been experimentally induced in the cat by electrical stimulation of the stellate ganglion [37]. Stimulation of the posterior hypothalamus produced extrasystoles that disappeared after ablation of these areas. Another site, the posterior corpora quadragemina and posterior portions of the cerebellum, when electrically stimulated resulted in multifocal premature ventricular contractions (PVC), nodal rhythm, and shifts of the SA sinoatrial node pacemaker. In their study, Greenshoot and Reichenbach stimulated the mesencephalic reticular formation in the cat and systematically produced elevation in systolic blood pressure, peaking of T waves, ST segment elevations, and arrhythmias in 50% of the animals [37]. Thus, experimental evidence demonstrates that many areas of the brain are capable of producing cardiovascular changes when stimulated by mechanical compression (as in increased ICP) or electrical current. The exact cause and effect relationship is similar, although evidence suggests that these stimuli, including local ischemia, do elicit elevations in plasma catecholamine levels with concurrent changes in cardiovascular parameters.

Myocardial damage may also occur. Creatine phosphokinase, myocardium brain (MB) isomer levels, and serial EKGs were evaluated in a group of severely head-injured patients [38]. All patients were comatose, had decerebrate or decorticate posturing, and were unresponsive to painful stimuli. All thirty patients demonstrated CPK elevations in one or more of the samples taken, with 93% having elevated MB concentrations. In contrast to the typical 24 to 36 hr elevation seen following myocardial infarction, the head-injured patients sustained elevations in the MB isomer for at least 3 days. The associated EKG changes included QT_c interval prolongation in twenty-seven of thirty patients and nonspecific ST-T wave changes in sixteen of thirty patients. Although one patient actually developed serial EKG changes and enzyme elevations consistent with myocardial infarction, no correlation could be found between CPK and MB activity and EKG changes and survival.

Histologic myocardial infarction changes in the myocardium of head-injured patients differ from those experiencing acute myocardial infarction in both area and distribution of damage. Following electrical stimulation of the midbrain reticular formation in the cat, scattered regions of myofibrillar degeneration are seen within the subendocardium accompanied by subendocardial hemorrhage. These changes are most prominent in the left ventricle around papillary muscle. Myocardial damage in acute head injury, as evidenced by autopsy reports, is distributed around nerve endings; those seen in acute myocardial infarction involve necrosis of all tissues supplied by the affected vessel [38]. Norepinephrine release around these myocardial nerve endings produces vasoconstriction and ischemia.

Catecholamine Secretion

Plasma catecholamine levels are significantly elevated after acute head injury. Plasma norepinephrine levels as high as 550 pg/ml (normal 250 pg/ml) have been recorded in patients sustaining severe head injury. A correlation also exists between decreasing GCS scores and plasma norepinephrine levels; a GCS less than 10 was associated with norepinephrine levels consistent with marked sympathetic nervous system activation and significant alterations in the hemodynamic state [39].

Such changes are reproducible in laboratory animals using techniques such as intracarotid injections of saline, induced blunt head trauma, induced cerebral ischemia, and intracisternal injections of veratrine and intravenous epinephrine. In one of the first experiments to demonstrate a temporal relationship between elevated ICP and catecholamine levels, Graf and Rossi produced extreme elevation in plasma catecholamine levels by placing an epidural balloon in the skull of dogs [40]. An initial 5 ml of saline injected into the balloon produced a transient ICP elevation of 150 to 200 mm Hg, lasting 3 to 4 sec. After spatial compensation occurred, ICP reverted to baseline only to become elevated and remain in the 80 to 160 mm Hg range after subsequent injections of 4 and 2 ml of saline. Accompanying these elevations were increases in systemic blood pressure and epinephrine, norepinephrine, and dopamine levels within 2.5 min. Epinephrine levels of 239 times normal baseline value were recorded along with less, but significant, increases in norepinephrine and dopamine [40].

A possible mechanism for these catecholamine increases has been proposed. Mechanical compression of the brain may stimulate the mesencephalon or medulla to release catecholamines. This response can be attenuated by transection of the cervical spinal cord, alpha-adrenergic blockade, or deep narcosis [41,42].

Therapy

Based on the assumption that catecholamine release from the injured brain affects cardiorespiratory function, appropriate pharmacologic intervention should decrease perioperative mortality and morbidity.

In planning such therapy one should be aware of the effects of drug therapy on cerebral blood flow (CBF) and ICP. The acutely head-injured patient frequently demonstrates impaired cerebral autoregulation or vasomotor paralysis. Any elevation in systemic blood pressure in this setting might therefore elevate CBF and ICP, causing cerebral edema. Blood pressure elevations greater than 30% of normal mean values should be treated with concurrent monitoring of ICP to ensure a cerebral perfusion pressure (CPP) of at least 80 mm Hg. Blood pressure has been controlled by use of beta-adrenergic blocking compounds or peripheral vasodilators. One might be falsely led to believe that a decrease in systemic blood pressure might be paralleled by a concurrent decrease in ICP. Keeping in mind the altered autoregulation in these patients, peripheral vasodilators such as sodium nitroprusside and hydralazine might not be the drugs of first choice. One study demonstrated a 20% reduction in systemic blood pressure accompanied by an 8% increase in CBF and 11% increase in ICP with the use of 5 to 15 mg of hydralazine intravenously. The ICP response occurred earlier than the systemic blood pressure reduction, indicating that the initial effect of hydralazine is on the cerebral capacitance vessels [43]. Sodium nitroprusside has been shown to have a similar effect in patients with intracranial mass lesions [44].

Beta-adrenergic blockade appears to be a better choice for management of hypertension and tachycardia. It has been shown to prevent the typical myocardial lesions produced in laboratory animals, and its role in limiting myocardial infarct size is well known [45]. Propranolol in increments totalling 1 to 4 mg, given slowly intravenously (over 5 min) is effective in slowing heart rate and lowering blood pressure without increasing ICP. In our institution we titrate propranolol to achieve a systolic blood pressure less than 160 mm Hg and diastolic blood pressure of less than 90 mm Hg. Decrease of heart rate to fewer than 70 beats per min is another useful end point [14]. Careful monitoring of blood pressure and ICP is required. Insertion of an arterial blood pressure monitor is routine in these patients. Adequate oxygenation and control of CPP are equally important in minimizing myocardial damage.

Continuous monitoring of ICP is extremely useful, especially when aggressive hyperventilation and diuretic therapy are employed. The ultimate effect of these therapeutic modalities on oxygen delivery to the brain is unknown because no direct measurement of CPP is available. Perhaps with the development of nuclear magnetic resonance (NMR) techniques, more useful guidelines in managing therapy will be available.

SUMMARY

The acutely head-injured patient is characterized by a hypoxic hyperdynamic cardiovascular state typified by decreased arterial saturation and elevations in heart rate, systemic blood pressure, and cardiac output. The most consistent EKG changes are prolongation of the QT_c interval and tall, peaked P waves. QT_c prolongation and pulmonary shunt over 15% have been associated with increased mortality.

Cardiorespiratory changes are most probably manifestations of significant elevations in plasma catecholamine levels caused by mechanical brain compression. Therapy requires adequate oxygenation, judicious use of beta-adrenergic blockade, and ICP control.

REFERENCES

1. Veith I, trans. The Yellow Emperor's classic of internal medicine. Berkeley: University of California Press, 1973;159–68.
2. Palmer SF, ed. The works of John Hunter, FRS, with notes. London: Longmann, Rees, 1835.
3. Lewin W. Changing attitudes to the management of severe head injuries. Br Med J 1976;1:1234–39.
4. Cannon WB. Cerebral pressure after trauma. Am J Physiol 1901;6:91–121.
5. Rose J, Valtonen S, Jennett B. Avoidable factors contributing to death after head injury. Br Med J 1977;2:615–18.
6. Frost EAM. Respiratory complications in neurological surgery. In Landolt AM ed. Prog Neurol Surg, Vol 11, Basel, Karger, 1983; 118–140.
7. Moss G, Staunton C, Stein AA. Cerebral etiology of the "shock lung syndrome." J Trauma 1972;12:885–90.
8. Weisman S. Edema and congestion of the lungs resulting from intracranial hemorrhage. Surgery 1939;6:772–79.
9. Theodore J, Robin ED. Pathogenesis of neurogenic pulmonary edema. Lancet 1975;2:749–51.
10. Neumann D, Bailey L. An overview of neurogenic pulmonary edema. J Neurosurg, Nursing 1980;12:206–09.
11. Moss G, Staunton C, Stein AA. The centrineurogenic etiology of the acute respiratory distress syndromes. Am J Surg 1971;126:37–40.
12. Miner ME, Kaufman HH, Graham SH. Disseminated intravascular coagulation and fiberolysis following head injury in children: frequency and prognostic implication. J Pediatr 1982;100:687–91.
13. Astrup T. Assay and content of tissue thromboplastin in different organs. Thromb Diath Haemonth 1965;14:401–16.
14. Miner ME, Allen SJ. Cardiovascular effects of severe head injury. In: Frost E, ed. Clinical anesthesia in neurosurgery. Boston: Butterworth, 1984;372.
15. Herndon JM. The syndrome of fat embolism. South Med J 1975;68:1577–84.
16. Plum F, Posner JB. The diagnosis of stupor and coma, 2nd ed. Philadelphia: F.A. Davis Co., 1972; 1–59.
17. Lee MC, Klassen AC, Heaney LM, Resch JA. Respiratory rate and pattern disturbances in acute brain stem infarction. Stroke 1976;78:382–85.
18. North JB. Abnormal breathing patterns associated with acute brain damage. Arch Neurol 1974;31:338–44.
19. Crockard HA, Coppel DC, Morrow WFK. Evaluation of hyperventilation in treatment of head injuries. Br Med J 1973;4:634–40.
20. Fouts JB, Brashear RE. Intermittent positive-pressure breathing. A critical appraisal. Postgrad Med 1976;59:103–07.
21. Wright FG, Jr., Foley MF, Downs JB, Hodges MR. Hypoxemia and hypocarbia following intermittent positive pressure breathing. Anesth Analg 1976;55:555–59.

22. Aidinis SJ, Shapiro HM, Van Horn K. Effects of positive end-expiratory pressure (PEEP) on intracranial pressure, sagittal sinus and cerebral perfusion pressures during experimental intracranial hypertension in the cat (abstract 58). Proc Am Assoc Neurol Surg April 1975.

23. Frost EAM. Effects of positive end-expiratory pressure on intracranial pressure and compliance in brain injured patients. J Neurosurg 1977;47:195–200.

24. Downs JB, Perkins HM, Modell JH. Intermittent mandatory ventilation. An evaluation. Arch Surg 1974;109:519–23.

25. Oberg PA, Sjostrand U. Studies of blood pressure regulation: III. Dynamics of arterial blood pressure in carotid sinus nerve stimulation. Acta Physiol Scan 1971;81:109.

26. Bunnel JB, Karlson KH, Shannon DC. High frequency positive pressure ventilation in dogs and rabbits (abstract). Am Rev Resp Dis 1978;117 (Suppl):289.

27. Bohn DJ, Miyasaka K, Marchak BE, Thompson WK, Froese AB, Bryan AC. Ventilation by high frequency oscillation. J Appl Physiol 1980;48:710–16.

28. Fukuchi Y, Roumos CS, Macklem PT. Convection, diffusion and cardiogenic mixing of inspired gas in the lung. An experimental approach. Respir Physiol 1976;26:77–90.

29. Butler WJ, Bohn DJ, Bryan AC. Ventilation by high frequency oscillation in humans. Anesth Analg 1980;59:577–84.

30. Todd MM, Tartant SM, Shapiro HM. The effects of high frequency positive pressure ventilation in intracranial pressure and brain surface movement in cats. Anesthesiology 1981;54:496–504.

31. Hamilton P, Orayemi B, Gillam J. Lung pathology following high frequency oscillation and conventional ventilation (abstract). Fed Proc 1982;41:1747.

32. Cushing H. Concerning a definite regulatory mechanism of the vasomotor center which controls blood pressure during cerebral compression. Johns Hopkins Hosp Bull 1901;12:290–92.

33. Clifton GL, McCormick WF, Grossman RG. Neuropathology of early and late deaths after head injury. Neurosurgery 1981;8:309–14.

34. Schulte am Esch J, Murday H, Pfeifer G. Haemodynamic changes in patients with severe head injury. Acta Neurochir 1980;54:243–50.

35. Brown RS, Mohr PA, Carey JS, Shoemaker WC. Cardiovascular changes after cranial cerebral injury and increased intracranial pressure. Surg Gyn Obstet 1967;125:1205–11.

36. Hersch C. Electrocardiographic changes in head injuries. Circulation 1961;23:853–60.

37. Greenshoot JH, Reichenbach DD. Cardiac injury and subarachnoid hemorrhage. A clinical pathological and physiologic correlation. J Neurosurg 1969;30:521–23.

38. Hackenberry LE, Miner ME, Rea GL, et al. Biochemical evidence of myocardial injury after severe head trauma. Crit Care Med 1982;10:641–44.

39. Clifton G, Ziegler M, Grossman R. Circulating catecholamines and sympathetic activity after head injury. Neurosurgery 1981;8:10–14.

40. Graf CJ, Rossi NP. Catecholamine response to intracranial hypertension. J Neurosurg 1978;49:862–68.

41. Chen HI, Sun SC, Chai CY. Pulmonary edema and hemorrhage resulting from cerebral compression. Am J Physio 1973;224:223–29.

42. Bean JW, Beckman DL. Centrogenic pulmonary pathology in mechanical head injury. J Appl Physiol 1969;27:807–12.

43. Ivergaard J, Skinhöj E. A paradoxical cerebral hemodynamic effect of hydralazine. Stroke 1975;6:402–404.
44. Cottrell J, Patel K, Ransahoff J, et al. Intracranial pressure changes induced by sodium nitroprusside in patients with intracranial mass lesions. J Neurosurg 1978;48:329–31.
45. Hunt D, Gore I. Myocardial lesions following experimental intracranial hemorrhages; prevention with propranolol. Am Heart J 1972;83/2:232–36.

Chapter 4

Management of Intracranial Hypertension

Steven J. Allen

One of the more significant contributions to the care of head-injured patients in recent years has been the recognition of the relationship between elevated intracranial pressure (ICP) and outcome. Miller et al [1] and, later, Saul and Ducker [2] demonstrated the striking difference in mortality when patients were classified by ICP. In the management of the patient with traumatic brain injury, the goals that have been established are to maintain the ICP below 20 mm Hg while the mean arterial pressure is at least 50 mm Hg higher. This pressure difference between the mean arterial pressure and the ICP is the cerebral perfusion pressure (CPP). These goals have resulted in the ICP's becoming a focus of therapy in and of itself. The protocols that have been devised for treatment of increased ICP have tended to assume that the cause of all ICP rises is the same; thus, elevated ICP results in a stereotypic therapeutic response [3,4]. This response fosters an attitude that, if the ICP is down, all is well. As is recognized, an ICP below 20 mm Hg may not result in an awake patient, and other pathologic processes may be occurring that are not reflected by an elevated ICP. A still greater concern arises from the therapy itself. Treatment that is focused on lowering the ICP may ultimately prove deleterious by resulting in insidious ischemia. Such ischemia may be undetected by ICP and CPP measurement. Thus, there is a need to monitor the effects of ICP treatment on cerebral oxygen delivery as such therapy may alter cerebral blood flow (CBF).

Elevated ICP after head injury is deleterious because it may interfere with cerebral perfusion and metabolism. Since the therapeutic goal is to maintain cerebral cellular integrity and prevent secondary injuries by providing the physiologic environment most conducive to recovery, ICP is only one important part of the approach to the treatment of patients with head injuries. ICP monitoring should foster an approach of differential diagnosis just as does any other physiologic measurement. The other pieces of information should include the general and neurologic exam, recent past history, cardiovascular and respiratory function, cerebral computerized tomography (CT), medications, and

41

as much data regarding cerebral blood flow (CBF) and metabolism as is available. We should be moving away from the use of a standard protocol directed at ICP to an orientation where intracranial hypertension requires as specific an etiologic diagnosis as possible. Therapy is then aimed at an identified cause. Processes other than brain swelling must be taken into account when the patient presents with an elevated ICP. The possible adverse effects of the ICP therapy must also be balanced against the benefits. Finally, we must begin to consider our therapy in terms of physiologic measurements other than ICP, particularly measures of CBF and metabolism. By replacing empiric therapy with guided therapy, better results may be achieved in this young population that is highly conducive to rehabilitation.

INTRACRANIAL COMPLIANCE

To understand the treatment of elevated ICP, the components of the intracranial vault need to be addressed. Intracranial contents consist of brain, blood, and cerebrospinal fluid (CSF). As expected, a rise in ICP is due to a rise in intracranial volume (ICV). In a rigidly enclosed fluid-filled space like the calvarium, one would expect volume and pressure increases to be linear. However, as indicated in Figure 4.1, the relationship is nonlinear. There appear to be effective compensatory mechanisms limiting a rise in ICP in the early part of the curve. Some explanations that have been advanced include shunting of CSF into the spinal canal and compression of the venous plexus. However, these mechanisms rather abruptly play out, with subsequent small rises in ICV leading to dramatic increases in ICP. The measurement of intracranial compliance can be performed by observing the ICP elevation after a given amount of saline, usually 1 cc or less, is injected through the ICP monitor. The determination of the compliance allows estimation of the patient's position on the curve and is probably a better indicator to follow than ICP alone, especially when the ICP is between 15 and 20 mm Hg [5].

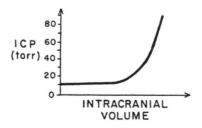

Figure 4.1   Intracranial compliance curve.

JUGULAR VENOUS PRESSURE

Once the compliance has decreased—i.e., the brain has become tight—attention to events that will further increase ICV is important. Since no valves exist in the venous system between the right atrium and the brain, central venous pressure elevations can be transmitted to the intracranial cavity and are reflected by undesirable ICP changes. Patients should be positioned in a 15 to 20° head-up tilt to enhance jugular venous outflow [6]. Placing these patients flat, as for a CT scan, can produce marked increases in ICP. Similarly, the head must be kept at midposition because lateral rotation of the head can occlude the ipsilateral internal jugular vein [7]. Care is taken not to place tape around the neck so that internal jugular drainage is not compromised. Although positive and expiratory pressure (PEEP) therapy theoretically could raise intrathoracic pressure and thereby have a deleterious effect on ICP, evidence suggests that PEEP levels up to 10 cm H_2O have little or no effect if the head of the bed and of the patient is elevated [8,9].

Activities found commonly in patients with head injuries such as posturing, breath holding, and tremors can lead to raised intrathoracic pressure and resultant elevated ICP [10]. For this reason, muscle relaxants are often used to reduce this cause of raised ICP.

CEREBRAL ARTERIOVENOUS OXYGEN DIFFERENCE

Much of conventional therapy probably has its major impact on ICP by manipulating the cerebral blood volume (CBV) via the CBF and perhaps the cerebral metabolic rate of oxygen ($CMRO_2$) [1] since CBV is related to CBF [11,12]. Cerebral oxygen delivery consists of the concentration of oxygen in the arterial blood (CaO_2) and the rate at which that blood is delivered to the brain (CBF). CBF represents a major determinant of cerebral oxygen delivery; thus, reductions in CBF, induced by therapy, have the potential of producing cerebral ischemia. Therefore, there is a need for a guide to cerebral hemodynamics in addition to CPP. The arterial-jugular venous oxygen content difference ($AJDO_2$) is a promising monitor of relative cerebral oxygen delivery in head injured patients.

The Fick equation restates the law of conservation of matter in biologic terms. If the total amount of oxygen leaving an organ is subtracted from that which is delivered, the result equals the amount of oxygen consumed. For the brain, this equation is:

$$CMRO_2 = CBF \times (CaO_2 - CjvO_2),$$

where $CMRO_2$ stands for cerebral metabolic rate of oxygen, CBF represents cerebral blood flow, and CaO_2 and $CjvO_2$ represent oxygen contents in ml per 100 ml blood of arterial and jugular venous blood respectively. Arterial oxygen content is readily sampled from any arterial site. Blood that is solely from the brain can be obtained by placing a catheter retrograde in the internal jugular vein (Figure 4.2) so the tip is in the superior portion of the jugular bulb [13]. Rearranging the Fick equation, we get:

$$\frac{CMRO_2}{CBF} = CaO_2 - CjvO_2 = AJDO_2$$

This expression shows how the arterial-jugular venous difference ($AJDO_2$) represents the ratio of $CMRO_2$ to CBF. The importance of this ratio is that regardless of the absolute cerebral oxygen consumption, the $AJDO_2$ reflects how appropriate global cerebral oxygen delivery is for the brain's current needs.

This ratio has practical and clinical relevance in the acute care of patients with closed head injuries. $CMRO_2$ cannot be measured directly but must be calculated. CBF is still somewhat difficult to reliably measure because a steady ICP, blood pressure, and $PaCO_2$ are required for at least 15 min. while the measurement is performed. In contrast, $AJDO_2$ requires only the measurement

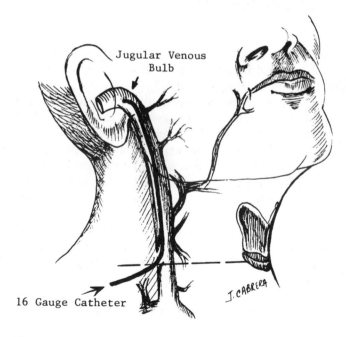

Figure 4.2   Position of jugular venous bulb catheter.

of the hemoglobin concentration and saturation of the arterial and jugular venous blood, which can be determined using an oximeter. The reproducibility of this measurement is excellent (1 to 2%). Since the arterial content does not change radically with CBF manipulations, it is the moment to moment changes in the jugular venous oxygen saturation that largely impacts the $AJDO_2$. If flow is decreased, then the brain will extract a greater percentage of the oxygen delivered as less total oxygen is supplied; that is, jugular venous oxygen tension will decrease, resulting in an increase in the $AJDO_2$.

Obrist et al have demonstrated a correlation between Glasgow Coma Scale score (GCS) and $CMRO_2$ [14]. It would appear that in closed head injuries, total cerebral oxygen consumption is related to how awake the patient is, regardless of the structural injury. Thus, if the patient's GCS is constant over an observation period, then the $CMRO_2$ has not changed and changes in the measured $AJDO_2$ reflect changes in CBF. $AJDO_2$ measurements from normal patients were published as part of Kety and Schmidt's initial work on CBF in 1948 [13]. Their value of 6.3 + 1.2 ml 02/100 ml blood has been confirmed by other studies. When cerebral oxygen delivery was decreased by hypotension in normal subjects, subjective evidence of cerebral ischemia developed at an $AJDO_2$ of approximately 9 ml 02/100 ml blood [15]. This value provides a maximum of $AJDO_2$ permissible in patients. However, perhaps a more appropriate upper limit of $AJDO_2$ would be 7.5 ml 02/100 ml blood, which is one standard deviation above the normal value. Assuming a PaO_2 of at least 70 mm Hg, a hemoglobin of 11 grams%, and a normal pH, an $AJDO_2$ of 7.5 ml 02/100 ml blood occurs when the jugular venous oxygen tension ($PjvO_2$) falls to 27 mm Hg. An $AJDO_2$ at this level or below, while maintaining an acceptable ICP, provides as optimal a cerebral hemodynamic environment for the injured brain as is currently possible.

$AJDO_2$ monitoring has at least two limitations. First, it is a global measurement, and regional areas of mismatched flow to consumption may not be detectable. However, Bruce and colleagues found that regional CBF (rCBF) appears to be relatively uniform following closed head injuries [16]. Even in areas of brain surrounding mass lesions, only rarely was rCBF significantly lower than in the rest of the brain. However, even if there are areas of heterogeneous flow to metabolism, a low jugular venous oxygen saturation must reflect possible ischemia somewhere in the brain. The use of $AJDO_2$ needs to be restricted to patients who have a diffuse injury, have not suffered a stroke, and do not have a large midline shift or other major focal abnormalities on cerebral CT.

The effect of alkalosis on the hemoglobal disassociation curve poses another problem. Alkalosis shifts the curve to the left (Bohr effect), resulting in lower partial pressure of oxygen for a given saturation of hemoglobin. This hemoglobin saturation shift has its major practical impact on the $CjvO_2$ and could cause the $AJDO_2$ to be less reliable in detecting ischemia when aggressive hyperventilation has resulted in profound respiratory alkalosis.

HYPERVENTILATION

Hyperventilation is an important means of lowering ICP because of the linear relationship between $PaCO_2$ and CBF [17–19]. There is a 3% decrease in CBF for every mm Hg drop in $PaCO_2$ between 200 and 70 mm Hg. Therefore, induced hypocapnia of 25–30 mm Hg results in a decrease of 25–30% in CBF. This reduction in a determinant of cerebral oxygen delivery is well tolerated in uninjured brains [18–20], but similar data are not documented for patients with head injuries. Recent evidence suggests that the underlying CBF in head injured patients can be quite variable and, therefore, the effect of routine hyperventilation on cerebral hemodynamics in the head injured is not uniform. Recognition that the CBF can be high or low has great implications on routine and empiric hyperventilation. Obrist et al [14] was able to divide their large series of head injured patients into two groups, based on whether the CBF was low or normal to high. In subjects with low CBF, coupling with $CMRO_2$ was found. ICP elevations were not as common a problem, and a subset of patients was identified who demonstrated suggestive ischemia during treatment with routine hyperventilation ($PaCO_2$ 25 to 30 mm Hg). In contrast, the second group had higher CBFs that were in excess of what would be expected and demonstrated no correlation of CBF to $CMRO_2$. A similar excess of flow to consumption was described in stroke models and termed luxury perfusion [21]. This group also developed more problems with ICP. As CO_2 responsiveness was still intact, this group would appear to benefit from further hypocapnia to bring the CBF to a level appropriate for the $CMRO_2$. The observation in this luxury perfusion group of a greater incidence of elevated ICP implicates the role of changes of CBF resulting in increased CBV and, thus, ICP. Knowledge of the ICP does not identify into which group a patient may fall. Calculation of the $AJDO_2$, however, estimates whether CBF is normalized to $CMRO_2$ and allows titration of hyperventilation to the patient's unique cerebral hemodynamic situation (Figure 4.3).

DIURETICS

Patients with head injuries may present with ICP elevation but $AJDO_2$ evidence suggestive of ischemia when hyperventilation is used. An appropriate treatment in this situation should include a therapy that does not decrease and possibly increases CBF while lowering ICP. Osmotic diuretics appear to be such agents [16]. The administration of mannitol may be helpful in reversing the development of ischemia by not decreasing CBF and effectively causing the ICP to fall. However, the use of mannitol when luxury perfusion exists may result in the enhancement of vasogenic edema. Although many clinical studies use mannitol, its exact mode of action as well as its effects on cerebral hemodynamics are unknown because of the rapid cerebral and systemic hemodynamic

AVDO2

WIDE	ISCHEMIA
NARROW	LUXURY PERFUSION

Figure 4.3 Significance of $AVDO_2$.

changes that take place with bolus injection. Further work in this area will require monitoring techniques that can track these very rapid changes.

HYPERTENSION

Cushing described the development of systemic arterial hypertension when ICP is progressively elevated [22]. Systemic arterial hypertension associated with the Cushing reflex is mediated by the sympathetic nervous system and represents an attempt to maintain cerebral perfusion. In such an instance, reduction in the systemic arterial blood pressure will result in a narrowing of the CPP to perhaps an ischemic level and produce potentially dangerous cerebral effects. When systemic arterial hypertension is a result of the Cushing reflex, the ICP rises first, approaching the arterial blood pressure, with subsequent rise of the latter.

Impaired autoregulation, in contrast, has been documented in a number of cerebral diseases, including head injury [23]. Autoregulation is the ability of cerebral arterioles to maintain a constant CBF across a wide spectrum of arterial pressures (normal—50 to 150 mm Hg). When the brain has sustained an injury, CBF becomes more pressure dependent. In these patients, when the blood pressure rises, either due to suctioning of the endotracheal tube, pain, etc., CBF rises and results in an increase in CBV and ICP. When intracranial compliance is low, that is, when the brain is tight, elevations in the systemic arterial blood pressure can be transmitted through the rest of the brain resulting in ICP elevation with a rise in CBF. ICP rises with or following the rise in blood pressure in these patients. Hyperventilation and mannitol are not as reasonable methods in managing these problems as are attempts to lower the blood pressure and/or to prevent its rise. In our experience, a variety of procedures such as posturing of the patient and tracheal suction are the most common causes of ICP elevations (unpublished data by the author). We recommend pretreatment of patients at risk with lidocaine 1 to 1.5 mg/kg IV 1 minute prior to suctioning, turning, or changing dressings. This dose of lidocaine has been found to attenuate the rise in blood pressure when given prior to suctioning [24]. Some patients will require narcotics as well as additional therapy prior to routine nursing care. We have found that in patients with poor intracranial compliance, the ICP is more easily controlled when pretreatment is given. There must be some concern for brief intermittent elevations of ICP, however, since these intermittent elevations may lead to transient hypoperfusion and ischemia, thereby worsening cerebral edema.

Attention must be given to the temporal relationship between the elevation in ICP and the hypertension. The treatment of hypertension induced ICP elevation has its own hierarchy for which a pathophysiologic basis will be established in the next section.

HYPERCATECHOLANEMIA

Head-injured patients frequently develop hypertension, tachycardia, and diaphoresis due to an increase in sympathetic activity. Clifton et al have characterized this hyperdynamic response in head-injured patients and implicated the autonomic nervous system as one possible route of mediation [25]. In fact, elevated catecholamines have been measured in a number of cerebral diseases, including head injuries. Norepinephrine and epinephrine levels have been reported to be three to five times normal in acute head injuries [26]. It would seem logical, then, to attempt to block the undesirable effects of these excessive catecholamines. Propranolol has been used with success in patients with closed head injuries [27] and is associated with an improved compliance when compared to the use of hydralazine. In patients with no history of heart disease or asthma, heart rate above 100, and a mean arterial pressure of greater than 100 mm Hg, we begin therapy with 1 to 2 mg IV and give 1 mg every 5 min until the heart rate is below 100. Large doses of propranolol may be required. These patients commonly require 8 to 10 mg in the first hour. If ICP control is improved, a continuous infusion of 1 to 2 mg/hr is started and titrated to keep the heart rate less than 100. A beta blocker is chosen because it directly blocks the cardiac catecholamine receptors with essentially no deleterious cerebral effects. Furthermore, if other hypotensive agents are required, dose requirements of such drugs will be reduced if the reflex tachycardia has been attenuated by beta blockade.

If adequate blood pressure control has not been achieved despite a slowing of the heart rate, more potent agents are indicated. A number of drugs such as sodium nitroprusside, trimethaphan, and nitroglycerin have been used in neuroanesthesia to induce hypotension [28,29]. Their use, however, in the normalization of hypertension in head-injured patients is less well documented.

A concern when the blood pressure is lowered in patients with elevated ICP is whether ischemia has developed because of the narrowed CPP. AJDO$_2$ monitoring becomes imperative when significant changes in CPP are anticipated. An illustrative case is shown in Table 4.1. This 32-year-old man suffered a closed head injury in a motor vehicle accident. He required prompt evacuation of bilateral epidural hematomas. Postoperatively, he was found to have a GCS of 6 with the vital signs listed. The amount of medication required to maintain

Table 4.1 Use of Trimethaphan in a 32-Yr-Old Man with Bilateral Epidural Hematomas and GCS Rating of 6 Following a Closed Head Injury

Physiologic Variables		Before Trimethaphan Begun	Trimethaphan Started
MAP	mm Hg	102	94
ICP	mm Hg	18	20
CPP	mm Hg	84	74
$PaCO_2$	mm Hg	27.5	28.8
$SjvO_2$	%	58	61
$AJDO_2$	ml O_2/100 cc blood	5.96	5.2
Total Rx required for 8 hours			
Morphine, mg		50	10
Metocurine, mg		30	10
Mannitol, gm		8.57	0

MAP: Mean arterial pressure
ICP: Intracranial pressure
CPP: Cerebral perfusion pressure
$SjvO_2$: Jugular venous oxygen saturation
$AJDO_2$: Arteriovenous oxygen difference

his ICP below 20 mm Hg for the 8 hours preceding antihypertensive therapy is listed in the left-hand column. Trimethaphan was titrated to lower his mean blood pressure by 10 mm Hg. This small reduction in blood pressure produced not only a marked reduction in medications for ICP control but also no $AJDO_2$ evidence of ischemia. Subsequently, tachyphylaxis developed and the blood pressure and ICP rose. Sodium nitroprusside was started with a similar beneficial response. The drug was able to be tapered over the next 2 days as the hypertension resolved. As the $AJDO_2$ did not change significantly with systemic arterial blood pressure manipulation, altered autoregulation probably was not a contributing cause to the ICP elevation. Most likely, transmission of the systemic arterial blood pressure was the main factor in this instance.

Although many authors have blamed adverse effects on cerebral vasodilation [28,29], no direct action of these drugs on the cerebral vasculature in humans has been convincingly demonstrated. The indirect evidence cited for the cerebral vasodilatory effects of sodium nitroprusside come from case reports in which the ICP rose as the blood pressure fell [28]. Indeed, Henrikson and Paulson infused sodium nitroprusside directly in the internal carotid artery of seven awake patients without any effect on CBF. When these same authors gave sodium nitroprusside systemically, they found a fall in CBF occurring when the blood pressure fell below the accepted lower limits of autoregulation [30]. Conceivably, the rise in ICP when the blood pressure was lowered might have been due to the ischemia that was produced but more likely it is the result of change in the cerebral vascular resistance. A study to measure the CBV, CBF, blood pressure, ICP, and $AJDO_2$ while the sodium nitroprusside is administered in head-injured patients would elucidate conflicting reports.

BARBITURATES

Barbiturates were first demonstrated to lower ICP in humans in 1937, a relatively short time after their introduction into clinical practice [31]. Their place, however, in the treatment of patients with closed head injuries remains controversial. In 1979, Marshall, Smith, and Shapiro published their results of its use in 100 patients suffering from head trauma. Twenty-five of these patients developed uncontrollable intracranial hypertension and were placed in barbiturate coma, 10 of whom made a good recovery [32]. This was hailed as a major advance in the care of the head injured and created much enthusiasm for this form of therapy. However, the study does not definitively answer the question of whether barbiturates alter the outcome from severe closed head injury. The study was not randomized and the percentage of patients with intractable intracranial hypertension was far greater than that reported by Miller et al [1] and reflected in our experience. Further, the incidence of intracranial hypertension intractable to conventional therapy reported by this same group was lower in subsequent studies [3,33]. To answer the question, the National Institutes of Health are sponsoring a multicenter randomized study of the effects of barbiturate coma on the outcome from head injuries. Our impression is that in cases where luxury perfusion exists in spite of hyperventilation, barbiturates are very effective, presumably by lowering CBF and $CMRO_2$ in parallel. When the $AJDO_2$ suggests ischemia, barbiturates still lower ICP but do not reverse the ischemia.

Currently barbiturate coma is used as a last resort in patients with intractable intracranial hypertension.

Induced barbiturate coma is essentially the process of placing a patient under general anesthesia. It requires an intensive care unit with a well-prepared staff, hemodynamic monitoring, and the ability to respond immediately to the many complex problems (including hypotension, ventilation, fluid balance, and recognition of subtle neurologic changes) commonly observed in these patients. If on maximal medical therapy the ICP is greater than 30 mm Hg for 30 min or 40 mm Hg for 5 min, and if an operable intracerebral lesion has been ruled out, barbiturate therapy should be started. Pentobarbital (15 mg/kg) is infused in the first hour as tolerated, closely monitoring the cardiac output and arterial pressure. Additional doses of pentobarbital 5 mg/kg are given over each of the next 3 hr, with 1 to 2 mg/kg/hr given as maintenance. Although blood levels can be helpful early in therapy, the demonstration of a 30 to 60 sec burst-suppression pattern on the electroencephalograph (EEG) has been correlated with maximal cerebral metabolic depression and may, therefore, be used as a monitor of effective dosing [34]. Obviously, much work needs to be done in this area to elucidate the appropriate role of barbiturates in the care of the head injured. However, it is unlikely that using ICP as a sole indicator for the use of barbiturates will be satisfactory.

ULTRASOUND

The supine position can be deleterious for head injured patients with low intracranial compliance. Unfortunately, modern CT scanners require this position to obtain a satisfactory study. Adding to this potential insult is the problem of transporting a critically ill patient to the radiology department. The patient's ICP is probably not going to be monitored as accurately, if at all, nor is the maintenance of hyperventilation and other aspects of the intensive care unit environment likely to be optimal. However, diagnosis and treatment of a surgically correctable lesion, such as a hematoma or hydrocephalus, is of great importance to the outcome of head-injured patients, making radiologic studies invaluable. At our institution, we have been placing a 1 × 3 cm burr hole at the time of ICP monitor placement. On the second postoperative day, after the scalp edema has been resolved, portable ultrasonography can be performed on a routine basis as a method of following a midline shift, the size of the ventricles, and/or the presence of hematomas. We believe this technique is a major addition to the improvement in the care of these patients. An example of how this technique has been used to detect the development of hydrocephalus in a patient with closed head injury is provided in Figure 4.4.

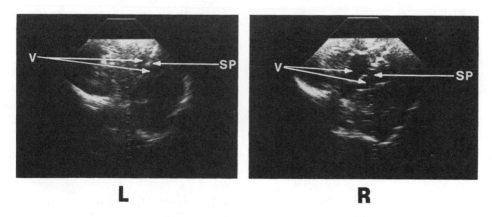

Figure 4.4   Ultrasound images through coronal burr hole made at time of admission. The image on the left was taken on the third postinjury day. The image on the right was taken some time later when clinical deterioration occurred. The ventricles are remarkably larger. V: ventricles; SP: septum pellucidum.

POSITRON EMISSION TOMOGRAPHY

The ideal therapy for head-injured patients is to provide every cell with adequate substrate for metabolism at an acceptable flow rate and pressure. Obviously, present techniques do not allow this kind of regional fine tuning. However, with the development of positron emission tomography (PET), it is now possible to measure regional flow and metabolism of oxygen and glucose in the brain. This research tool offers exciting promise in defining treatment regimens more clearly. However, even though PET scanning will add invaluable information to our understanding of cerebral metabolism and flow in the head injured, expense and availability factors will demand the use of simple and inexpensive bedside techniques such as $AJDO_2$ and ICP monitoring.

SUMMARY

We have emphasized the importance of differential diagnosis when planning therapy for elevated ICP and have presented diagnostic techniques for choosing the appropriated course. $AJDO_2$ monitoring and portable cerebral ultrasonography have been put forth as simple bedside tools for gaining additional information. The overall goal in the care of all critically ill patients is to provide every injured cell with adequate substrate to encourage recovery. Although most of our current methods of monitoring the injured brain are global, continuous monitoring of regional intracranial metabolism and flow combined with therapies that allow manipulation of these variables on a local basis represent the next level of treatment in the future.

REFERENCES

1. Miller JD, Becker DP, Ward JD, Sullivan HG, Adams WE, Rosner MJ. Significance of intracranial hypertension in severe head injury. J Neurosurg 1977;47:503–16.
2. Saul TG, Ducker TB. Effect of intracranial pressure monitoring and aggressive treatment on mortality in severe head injury. J Neurosurg 1982;56:498–503.
3. Marshall LF, Bowers SA. Medical management of intracranial pressure. In: Cooper PR, ed. Head injury. Baltimore: Williams and Wilkins, 1982; Chapter 9, 129–46.
4. Miller JD. Barbiturates and raised intracranial pressure. Ann Neurol 1979;6:189–93.
5. Miller JD, Leech P. Effects of mannitol and steroid therapy on intracranial volume-pressure relationships in patients. J Neurosurg 1975;42:274–81.
6. Durward QJ, Amacher L, Del Maesstro RF, Sibbald WJ. Cerebral and cardiovascular responses to changes in head elevation in patients with intracranial hypertension. J Neurosurg 1983;59:938–44.
7. Marsh ML, Marshall LF, Shapiro HM. Neurosurgical intensive care. Anesthesiology 1977;17:149–63.

8. Frost EAM. Effects of positive end-expiratory pressure on intracranial pressure and compliance in brain-injured patients. J Neurosurg 1977;47:195–200.

9. Arbushi W, Herkt G, Speckner E, Birk M. The effect on ICP of PEEP—ventilation and elevation of the upper body in patients with cerebral injuries. Anaesthetist 1980;29:521–24.

10. Shapiro HM. Intracranial hypertension: therapeutic and anesthetic considerations. Anesthesiology 1975;43:445–71.

11. Kuhl DE, Alavi A, Hoffman EJ, Phelps ME, Zimmerman RA, Obrist WD, Bruce DA, Greenberg JH, Uzzell B. Local cerebral blood volume in head-injured patients. J Neurosurg 1980;52:309–20.

12. Grubb RL, Jr., Raichle ME, Eichling JO, Ter-Pogossian MM. The effects of changes in $PaCO_2$ on cerebral blood volume, blood flow, and vascular mean transit time. Stroke 1974;5:630–39.

13. Kety SS, Schmidt CF. The nitrous oxide method for the quantitative determination of cerebral blood flow in man: theory, procedure and normal values. J Clin Invest 1948;27:476–83.

14. Obrist WD, Langfitt TW, Jaggi JL, Cruz J, Gennarelli TA. Cerebral blood flow and metabolism in comatose patients with acute head injury. J Neurosurg 1984;61:241–53.

15. Finnerty FA, Jr., Witkin L, Fazekas J. Cerebral hemodynamics during cerebral ischemia induced by acute hypotension. J Clin Invest 1954;33:1227–32.

16. Bruce D, Langfitt TW, Miller JD, Schutz H, Vapalahti MP, Stanek A, Goldberg HI. Regional cerebral blood flow, intracranial pressure, and brain metabolism in comatose patients. J Neurosurg 1973;38:131–44.

17. Crockard HA, Coppel DL, Morrow WFK. Evaluation of hyperventilation in treatment of head injuries. Br Med J 1973;4:634–40.

18. Kety SS, Schmidt CF. The effects of altered arterial tensions of carbon dioxide and oxygen on cerebral blood flow and cerebral oxygen consumption of normal young men. J Clin Invest 1948;27:484–91.

19. Raichle ME, Posner JB, Plum F. Cerebral blood flow during and after hyperventilation. Arch Neurol 1970;23:394–403.

20. Wollman H, Smith TC, Stephen GW, Colton ET III, Gleaton HE, Alexander SC. Effects of extremes of respiratory and metabolic alkalosis on cerebral blood flow in man. J Appl Physiol 1968;24:60–65.

21. Lassen NA. The luxury-perfusion syndrome and its possible relation to acute metabolic acidosis localized within the brain. Lancet 1966;ii:1113–15.

22. Cushing H. Concerning a definite regulatory mechanism of the vaso-motor centre which controls blood pressure during cerebral compression. Johns Hopkins Hosp Bull 1901; September:290–94.

23. Baldy-Moulinier M, Frerebeau P. Cerebral blood flow in cases of coma following severe head injury. In: Brock M, Fieschi C, Ingvar DH, Lassen NA, Schurmann K, eds. Cerebral blood flow. Berlin: Springer-Verlag, 1969:216–18.

24. Donegan MF, Bedford RF. Intravenously administered lidocaine prevents intracranial hypertension during endotracheal suctioning. Anesthesiology 1980;52:516–18.

25. Clifton GL, Robertson CS, Kyper K, Taylor AA, Dhekne RD, Grossman RG. Cardiovascular response to severe head injury. J Neurosurg 1983;59:447–54.

26. Clifton GL, Ziegler MG, Grossman RG. Circulating catecholamines and sympathetic activity after head injury. Neurosurgery 1981;8:10–14.

27. Robertson CS, Clifton GL, Taylor AA, Grossman RG. Treatment of hypertension associated with head injury. J Neurosurg 1983;59:455–60.
28. Turner JM, Powell D, Gibson RM, McDowall DG. Intracranial pressure changes in neurosurgical patients during hypotension induced with sodium nitroprusside or trimethaphan. Br J Anaesth 1977;49:419–25.
29. Cottrell JE, Gupta B, Rappaport H, Turndorf H, Ransohoff J, Flamm ES. Intracranial pressure during nitroglycerin-induced hypotension. J Neurosurg 1980;53:309–11.
30. Henriksen L, Paulson OB. The effects of sodium nitroprusside on cerebral blood flow and cerebral venous blood gases. Eur J Clin Invest 1982;12:389–93.
31. Horsley SJ. Intracranial pressure during barbital narcosis. Lancet 1937;1:141–43.
32. Marshall LF, Smith RW, Shapiro HM. The outcome with aggressive treatment in severe head injuries. Part II: acute and chronic barbiturate administration in the management of head injury. J Neurosurg 1979;50:26–30.
33. Bowers SA, Marshall LF. Outcome in 200 consecutive cases of severe head injury treated in San Diego County: a prospective analysis. Neurosurgery 1980;6:237–42.
34. Kassell NF, Hitchon PW, Gerk MK, Martin DS, Hill TR. Alterations in cerebral blood flow, oxygen metabolism, and electrical activity produced by high dose sodium thiopental. Neurosurgery 1980;7:598–603.

Chapter 5

Modulating Cerebral Oxygen Delivery and Extraction in Acute Traumatic Coma

Julio Cruz
Michael E. Miner

Cerebral hemodynamic and metabolic factors have been extensively studied under normal circumstances and in a variety of animal models and human pathologic conditions. Normal values from human volunteers for cerebral oxygen extraction have been available for over 40 years [1]. However, it was not until blood flow was adequately quantified that total cerebral consumption of oxygen and glucose could be measured. The landmark contribution of Kety and co-workers in the measurement of cerebral blood flow (CBF) and cerebral oxygen consumption ($CMRO_2$) in normal human volunteers provided researchers the opportunity to study further cerebral hemodynamics and metabolism [2].

Later, Guillaume [3] and Lundberg [4] demonstrated that intracranial pressure (ICP) could be safely measured for prolonged periods of time and in critically ill patients. Subsequently, the hemodynamic factors influencing intracranial hypertension were widely studied, and major contributions came from a variety of sources. However, Langfitt and co-workers derived significant information from animal studies that was extrapolated clinically [5,6]. Especially important were the data containing cerebral vasomotor paralysis.

In acute brain trauma, studies on cerebral hemodynamics and metabolism have added substantially to a comprehensive view of the multiple pathophysiologic variables affecting ICP [7–13]. Although intracranial hemorrhage and cerebral edema are currently felt to be important mechanisms in the development of severely increased ICP, they are not the exclusive cause of increased ICP after brain trauma. An increase in intracranial blood volume, cerebral hypervolemia, has been elegantly demonstrated with modern imaging techniques in an animal model of intracranial hypertension [14]. In some instances, cerebral hypervolemia also appears to be a significant treatable cause of increased ICP in head-injured patients.

In the most acute phase after injury, adult comatose patients have reduced $CMRO_2$ [11,15]. However, CBF is not as predictable and may be increased, decreased, or normal. A concomitant reduction of CBF when $CMRO_2$ is decreased reflects preservation of the metabolic flow matching. Conversely, normal or increased CBF in the face of decreased $CMRO_2$ reflects a relative or absolute cerebral hyperemia and a degree of metabolism flow mismatch.

Estimates of global $CMRO_2$/CBF matching are provided by measuring oxygen extraction parameters:

The arterial-jugular bulb oxygen content differences:

$$AJDO_2 = CaO_2 - CjO_2$$

The O_2 extraction fraction:

$$(O_2EF = AJDO_2/CaO_2)$$

By definition:

$$AJDO_2 = CMRO_2/CBF$$

Inspection of this equation reveals that relative to unknown levels of consumption, hypo- and hyperperfusion will be reflected, respectively, by high or low $AJDO_2$ (and O_2EF) values. If consumption ($CMRO_2$) is constant between measurements, changes in flow will be represented by inverse but proportionate changes in extraction.

It was not in brain-injured patients that these relationships were first demonstrated but in awake people sustaining acute reductions in systemic arterial pressure (SAP). These studies provided clear evidence that $CMRO_2$ can be maintained by increasing oxygen extraction to compensate for reductions in oxygen delivery due to reduced CBF [16,17]. Of particular importance in those studies was the correlation of clinical signs of cerebral ischemia (oligemic hypoxia) with critically low CBF and proportionately increased $AJDO_2$ values. Also, in awake humans, profound hypocapnia resulted in clinical signs of cerebral ischemia and electroencephalograph (EEG) abnormalities that were associated with jugular oxygen tensions comparable to the preceding $AJDO_2$ values [18]. Thus, the extraction parameters can be utilized to monitor the sufficiency of blood flow needed to maintain cerebral metabolic consumption. This concept is of paramount importance in deeply comatose patients, in whom a critically low CBF cannot be estimated by neurologic signs.

Hyperventilation is a potent method of lowering ICP in the acutely head-injured patient. However, approximately half these patients have reduced blood flow that cannot be determined by ICP monitoring, clinical examination, or standard brain-imaging techniques. Indeed, $AJDO_2$ monitoring can provide a method of determining whether hyperventilation is decreasing CBF to oligemic levels [11,19]. Similarly, $AJDO_2$ monitoring can be utilized to modulate CBF relative to $CMRO_2$ under a variety of therapeutic regimens. This allows a rapid assessment of treatment efficacy and places therapeutic decisions on a more rational basis.

To evaluate the clinical utility of serial $AJDO_2$ monitoring in acutely brain-injured patients, measurements were correlated with the initial findings on computed tomography (CT) of the brain, Glasgow Coma Scale (GCS) score, cerebral perfusion pressure (CPP = mean SAP − ICP), and arterial PCO_2. Observations were also made on the effects of physiologic and therapeutic interventions on these variables [20]. We found that $AJDO_2$ provided information about the matching of $CMRO_2$ to CBF that was not as clear from CBF measurements alone. Figure 5.1 illustrates the data from a patient whose admission brain CT revealed a small right frontal hemorrhagic contusion. ICP was kept in the normal range with moderate hypocapnia. At 9 hours a CBF measurement revealed a low flow, but resuming hyperventilation did not induce

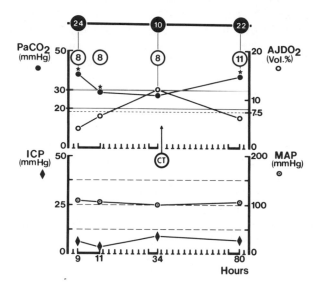

Figure 5.1　Serial $AJDO_2$ monitoring in two patients. $PaCO_2$, ICP, $AJDO_2$, and mean SAP (MAP) plotted against hours from injury. In the upper panel, closed-circled numbers along the heavy horizontal line are mean CBF values (given in ml/100 gm/min) averaged from sixteen external detectors, eight over each hemisphere (intravenous ^{133}Xe technique), and open-circled numbers are GCS scores from shortly before the measurements. In the $PaCO_2$ scale, 20 to 30 corresponds to the usual range of hyperventilation. In the $AJDO_2$ scale, 7.5 corresponds to 1 S.D. (standard deviation) above the normal mean. Stars indicate $PaCO_2$ values obtained after intentional ventilatory changes. Circled CT indicates repeat brain CT scan; circled m indicates mannitol 25% intravenous bolus of 12.5 gm; circled Bg indicates additional hyperventilation by bagging.

This patient represents the effect of an intracerebral hemorrhage on $AJDO_2$. Descriptions appear in the text.

oligemic hypoxia. A left hemiparesis gradually developed over the next day but with no change in the GCS. A repeat CBF measurement showed a further decrease while $CMRO_2$ was virtually unchanged because the $AJDO_2$ nearly doubled. A repeat CT revealed a delayed right frontal intracerebral hematoma. After removal of the hematoma, CBF was still reduced but was coupled with $CMRO_2$ with a normal $AJDO_2$. This patient represents matching of oxygen delivery and utilization in the face of decreased total cerebral blood flow. On the other hand, the data represented in Figure 5.2 is of a patient whose admission CT was unremarkable except for a small nonhemorrhagic contusion. The ICP was easily controlled by standard hyperventilation. At 13 hours, CBF and $AJDO_2$ indicated a mild cerebral hyperemia. Following a period of spontaneous $AJDO_2$ reduction (16 to 21 hours), ICP problems developed but further hyperventilation successfully offset the hyperemia. After another 24 hours of normal and stable ICP recordings (67 to 91 hours), the patient was slowly weaned to P_aCO_2 levels of over 30 mm Hg, while ICP and $AJDO_2$ remained in the normal range. This case illustrates the benefit of further hyperventilation in a patient with mild hyperemia. The ease with which the $AJDO_2$ data were obtained revealed the method to be more practical and less time consuming, as well as less expensive and more easily repeatable, than any currently available CBF technique.

We have now monitored $AJDO_2$ serially in over 150 severely head-injured patients with very gratifying results. However, factors in addition to flow-related changes in O_2 delivery and extraction appeared to be playing a role when clinical and/or physiologic deterioration was noted in some patients. Occasionally arterial oxygenation was noted to change in severely head-injured patients for no clear reason. Therefore, to enhance our monitoring capabilities, we felt it appropriate and desirable to evaluate continuous oxygen monitoring. Fortunately, currently available continuous oximetry does allow oxygen saturation to be monitored intravascularly [21,22]. This chapter records our current experience in continuous $AJDO_2$ monitoring in which we attempted to modulate not only global CBF but also arterial oxygen content (CaO_2).

CLINICAL MATERIAL AND METHODS

Patient Selection

Sixteen comatose adults, ranging in age from 16 to 67 years, were prospectively evaluated. There were thirteen males and all patients were reportedly healthy prior to injury. All patients had nonpenetrating, acute brain injuries with predominantly diffuse findings on CT scan. GCS scores on hospital admission were 4, 5, or 6 in fourteen cases. Two patients had GCS scores of 7 because of unilateral localizing motor responses even though they had pathologic posturing on the contralateral side. In the four cases with emergency surgery, the dura was closed in a watertight fashion, and bone flaps were returned to their

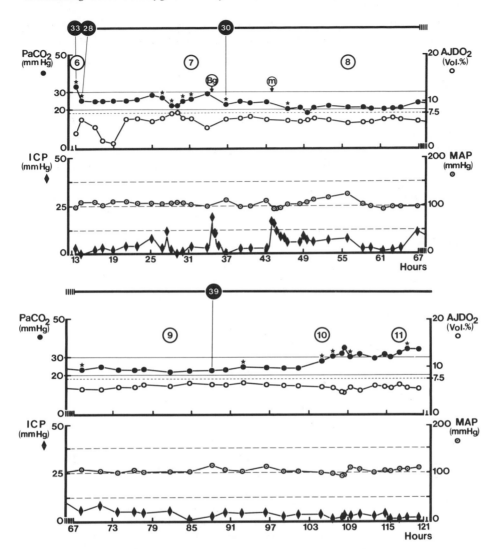

Figure 5.2 Serial $AJDO_2$ monitoring in two patients. $PaCO_2$, ICP, $AJDO_2$, and mean SAP (MAP) plotted against hours from injury. In the upper panel, closed-circled numbers along the heavy horizontal line are mean CBF values (given in ml/100 gm/min) averaged from sixteen external detectors, eight over each hemisphere (intravenous ^{133}Xe technique), and open-circled numbers are GCS scores from shortly before the measurements. In the $PaCO_2$ scale, 20 to 30 corresponds to the usual range of hyperventilation. In the $AJDO_2$ scale, 7.5 corresponds to 1 S.D. (standard deviation) above the normal mean. Stars indicate $PaCO_2$ values obtained after intentional ventilatory changes. Circled CT indicates repeat brain CT scan; circled m indicates mannitol 25% intravenous bolus of 12.5 gm; circled Bg indicates additional hyperventilation by bagging.

This patient represents the effect of an intracerebral hemorrhage on $AJDO_2$. Descriptions appear in the text.

anatomic position and held in place with wire sutures. Table 5.1 summarizes the major findings on the admission brain CTs of these sixteen patients.

Monitoring Features

After emergency CT brain imaging was performed, all patients went to the operating room for placement of an ICP monitoring device and craniotomy if needed. Once in the surgical intensive care unit, continuous electronic monitoring of SAP and ICP was performed. In patients requiring more careful fluid management, cardiac output and pulmonary arterial blood gases were monitored in addition to routine arterial blood gases.

Supplemental monitoring consisted of continuously recorded femoral arterial and jugular bulb oxyhemoglobin percent saturation by 4 Fr fiberoptic oximetry catheters, each connected to an optical module and signal processor (Oximetrix, Inc.). Expired CO_2 (P_ECO_2) was also continuously monitored from the endotracheal tube. The analog output from the SAP, P_ECO_2, ICP, SaO_2,

Table 5.1 Summary of Major Findings on the Admission Brain CT Scans in the Sixteen Cases

Case no.	SAH	SDH	CNT	ESM	UPC	BPC	DAI
1				x	x		
2	x		x				
3	x		x	x	x		x
4	x		x	x	x		x
5	x		x				
6			x	x		x	
7	x	x *	x	x	x		
8			x	x			x
9	x	x	x	x			
10	x	x *	x	x		x	
11			x	x			
12	x		x				
13	x	x *	x	x	x		
14	x		x	x			
15	x		x	x	x		
16	x		x	x	x		
Totals	12	4	15	13	7	2	3

SAH: Subarachnoid hemorrhage
SDH: Subdural hematoma
CNT: Contusions (hemorrhagic and/or nonhemmorhagic)
ESM: Effacement of sulcal markings (hemispheral and/or diffuse)
UPC: Unilateral obliteration of the perimesencephalic cistern
BPC: Bilateral obliteration of the perimesencephalic cistern
DAI: Deep white matter hemorrhages suggestive of diffuse axonal injury
Asterisk indicates significant shift of midline structures, over 5 mm.

and oxygen saturation in the jugular vein (SjO_2) monitors were converged to a variable speed strip chart recorder. This supplemental monitoring was initiated between 6 and 34 hr after injury (less than 24 hr in fourteen of the sixteen cases). SO_2 values from conventional oximetry were routinely used for in vivo calibration of the on-line SO_2 monitors.

Monitoring was discounted if ICP recordings were no longer required (thirteen cases), if there were technical difficulties (at 2 and 14 day in two cases), or if the patient expired (one case). The cumulative supplemental monitoring time was over 2,660 hr in the sixteen patients. A further 650 hr of SaO_2 monitoring was performed in eight of these patients who had prolonged pulmonary complications, thus requiring additional surveillance for arterial hypoxemia.

Blood samples from both the femoral artery (153 samples) and jugular bulb (151 samples) were analyzed by conventional oximetry in thirteen patients and compared to the indwelling fiberoptic oximetry catheter values. Correlations were assessed by linear regression analysis.

AJDO$_2$, Oligemic and Hypoxemic Hypoxia

For this investigation, we adopted norms from Gibbs and co-workers [1]. Normal values are 6.7 + 1.6 vol% for $AJDO_2$, 93.9 + 2% for SaO_2, and 61.8 + 7.4% for SjO_2 [mean and 2 SD (standard deviations)]. Abnormally low values were graded as follows:

Grade I	SaO_2 = 86 to 90%	SjO_2 = 50 to 54%
Grade II	SaO_2 = 81 to 85%	SjO_2 = 45 to 49%
Grade III	SaO_2 > 81%	SjO_2 > 45%

Oligemic and hypoxemic events were defined as early if they occurred within the first 72 hr after monitoring was initiated or late if after that time. Brief episodes lasted up to 10 min, and prolonged episodes were those lasting longer than 10 min. The duration of hypoxic events primarily reflects the length of time it took for their successful management. Several brief episodes were incompletely documented and were therefore excluded from analysis.

Cumulative Treatment Protocol

The protocol for ICP control below 20 mm Hg consisted of nine modalities used in a cumulative fashion:

Sedation (morphine sulfate),
Muscle paralysis (metubine iodide),

Hyperventilation to SjO_2 values no lower than 50 to 54%,

Hypertonic (25%) mannitol boluses to a serum osmolality no greater than 315 mOsm,

Cerebrospinal fluid (CSF) drainage,

Barbiturate coma (pentobarbital sodium),

Hypothermia,

Hypertonic mannitol boluses regardless of osmolality,

Decompressive craniotomy.

This protocol was followed in all cases, and progression of treatment defined severe intracranial hypertension (SICH).

Intracranial Hypertension

The first three steps of the cumulative treatment protocol were usually combined for the initial management of increased ICP. Patients were subsequently classified as having SICH if further therapeutic steps were required to maintain ICP less than 20 mm Hg for periods greater than 24 hr.

Relation to Neurologic Status

Changes in neurologic status were monitored by GCS scores and correlated with ICP and episodes of oligemic and/or hypoxemic hypoxia. Two patients were excluded from the final analysis because of prolonged barbiturate-induced coma for the treatment of SICH. Because half the patients underwent isolated SaO_2 monitoring for prolonged periods of time, GCS changes following hypoxemic events were analyzed in terms of decreases in SaO_2 both during periods of SICH and after ICP problems had subsided.

RESULTS

Correlation with Conventional Oximetry

SaO_2 values were in excellent agreement with the fiberoptic measurements ($n = 153$, $r = .98$). Overall, the correlation between SaO_2 values was much better than that of SjO_2 ($n = 151$, $r = .79$). However, by comparing light intensity tracings, we were able to identify two subsets of SjO_2 measurements: From periods of stable recordings a good correlation was found ($n = 122$, $r = .90$), while unstable recordings, demonstrated by the presence of dots in place of intensity tracings, yielded poorly correlated values ($n = 29$, $r = .68$). The most common source of recording instability was inadequate positioning of the patient's neck during passive postural changes, a relatively frequent problem encountered in the preliminary phase of this investigation.

Early Monitoring Findings and Management

When supplementary monitoring was initiated, all patients were being moderately or markedly hyperventilated for ICP control. In fifteen cases CPP was in the range of 60 mm Hg or higher with ICP below 20 mm Hg in fourteen of them. Only one case had CPP below 60 mm Hg. All patients had normal SaO_2, and fourteen presented with moderate degrees of respiratory alkalosis. Nine patients were in the oligemic category, and four of them (25%) were grade III (Table 5.2).

Excluding two patients in whom barbiturate loading preceded supplemental monitoring, those with ICP of less than 20 mm Hg and normal CPP, associated with SjO_2 values in the range of 55% or higher, were maintained in the same treatment modality until changes in CPP, SaO_2, and/or SjO_2 indicated a need for further therapy. Those with oligemia were managed with a combination of PCO_2 increases and/or intravenous mannitol boluses, depending on their baseline ICP levels. Patients with ICP recordings close to 20 mm Hg, associated with oligemia, were treated primarily with mannitol. Subsequent ICP reductions, if still accompanied by oligemic changes, were managed by raising PCO_2 to raise CBF physiologically. As expected, repeat mannitol

Table 5.2 Summary of Initial Monitoring Findings in the Sixteen Cases

Case no.	ICP <10	ICP 10-20	ICP >20	CPP <60	CPP 60-80	CPP >80	PCO2 <20	PCO2 20-25	PCO2 26-30	SjO2 <45	SjO2 45-54	SjO2 >54
1	x					x		E	A		x	
2		x			x			E A				x
3		x			x		E	A			x	
4		x				x		E A		x		
5		x				x	E	A				x
6		x			x			E A			x	
7		x				x	E	A				x
8		x			x			E	A		x	
9			x		x		E	A				x
10			x	x			E A				x	
11	x				x			E A			x	
12		x				x		E	A			x
13		x			x		E	A			x	
14		x			x			E	A		x	
15	x					x			E A			x
16		x			x			E	A			x

Note: E means expired PCO_2, and A means arterial PCO_2.

boluses were frequently required for ICP control after PCO_2 rises. Nonoligemic cases, with elevated ICP, were primarily treated with hyperventilation, which was gradually maximized, depending on SjO_2 allowances. Figure 5.3 illustrates the data obtained over 4 minutes after mannitol was given to a patient with CT evidence of diffuse brain swelling, multiple hemorrhagic contusions, diffuse axonal injury, and subarachnoid hemorrhage. Because the ICP was about 20 mm Hg and $PECO_2$ could not be safely increased, mannitol was given. This resulted in a partial reversal of the oligemia and suggests a direct effect of mannitol on cerebral blood flow and oxygen extraction.

Reversal of Oligemic Changes

Eight cases were found to have oligemia despite normal CPP within an hour after the jugular bulb catheter was inserted. The combination of mannitol and

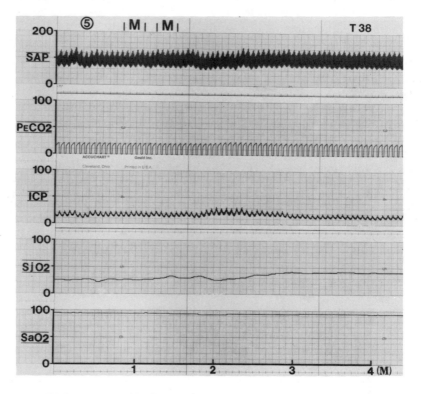

Figure 5.3 SAP, P_ECO_2, ICP, SjO_2, and SaO_2 recorded against minutes. Along the top, open-circled number is the GCS score from shortly before the recording period. M is mannitol 25% intravenous bolus of 12.5 gm; T is patient's rectal temperature (degrees Celsius). This figure represents the effect of mannitol on CBF and oxygen extraction.

PCO_2 manipulations effectively increased critically low SjO_2 values while allowing CPP to be maintained at adequate levels. Only one of these cases had spontaneous and recurrent oligemia. This case, illustrated in Figure 5.3, required larger amounts of mannitol than the others because ICP increases precluded further PCO_2 increases to allow increases in CBF. A ninth patient developed an initial decrease in CPP to oligemic levels due to an ominous combination of arterial hypotension, marked SICH, and additional hemodynamic instability associated with barbiturate loading. These findings were ultimately complicated by severe sepsis, leading to his death.

Thus, in the early monitoring phase (72 hr), oligemia was reversible while maintaining satisfactory CPP. In four of the sixteen patients, transient oligemia was caused either by mannitol boluses given to lower ICP (Figure 5.4) or by attempts to maximize hypocapnia. These transient oligemic episodes excluded, fifteen of the patients presented with either normal or narrow $AJDO_2$ for most of the acute phase—that is, from the start of monitoring in seven, and after reversing the oligemia in eight. In sharp contrast to managing the early oligemia, whenever delayed $AJDO_2$ narrowing was associated with intracranial

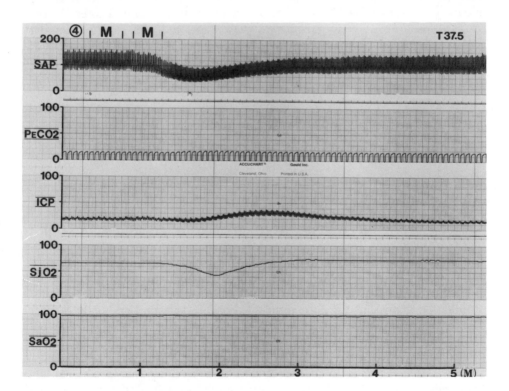

Figure 5.4 Recordings from a patient with diffuse brain swelling illustrating a fall in arterial blood pressure after two mannitol boluses. The associated decrease in SjO_2 suggests an autoregulatory defect.

hypertension, hyperventilation could very frequently be successfully utilized as a management technique.

Hypoxemia

Fifteen of the patients had continuous SaO_2 monitoring for as long as 2 wk. Eighty-six well-documented hypoxemic episodes were recorded. Sixty-three of these hypoxemic events occurred in association with well-defined, untoward ventilatory, pulmonary, and/or hemodynamic events, while the remaining twenty-three episodes were not associated with a definable cause. Fifty-three episodes, twenty-two of unclear etiology, occurred within the first 72 hr in thirteen of the patients. In contrast, only one of the thirty-three late hypoxemic episodes was not associated with definable pulmonary complications. That one event occurred immediately after an acute increase in ICP. Sixty-four of these hypoxic events were short lived (responded promptly to treatment), while twenty-two were prolonged (did not promptly respond to treatment). Of the short-lived events, twenty-two (34%) were not associated with definable causes. In contrast, all prolonged events except one were associated with severe pulmonary complications, mainly pneumonia, often combined with hemodynamic instability. That single exception was related to an error in the alarm system that resulted in a prolonged hypoxic event going undetected.

Half the patients had prolonged hypoxic episodes. Two were grade I and six were grades II and III events. Brief and prolonged episodes were nearly evenly distributed in the early and late monitoring stages.

Intracranial Hypertension

The first three therapeutic modalities of the cumulative treatment protocol (sedation, muscle paralysis, and hyperventilation) were sufficient for adequate ICP control in only two patients. The remaining fourteen patients were categorized as having SICH because they required more treatment than sedation, paralysis, and hyperventilation for longer than 24 hr. Ten of these fourteen did not have surgical mass lesions. Three patients did have emergency craniotomies on admission for evacuation of an acute subdural and/or intraparenchymal hematoma, and one additional patient had a partial frontal lobectomy 48 hr after admission because of refractory SICH.

Of the fourteen patients with SICH, mannitol boluses were sufficient as a final measure to control ICP in eight. Of the remaining six patients, five underwent periodic CSF drainage, which served as a final step in three. The sixth case, who had a subarachnoid bolt instead of an ICP monitoring catheter, went from mannitol to barbiturate coma, along with the two in whom CSF drainage was not sufficient. One of these patients expired, one went on to require frontal lobectomy, and barbiturates ameliorated the SICH in the third.

Relation to Neurologic Status

Oligemic changes were promptly reversed in seven of nine patients. Induced barbiturate coma on the first day post injury precluded an adequate neurologic examination in two patients with SICH. This limited discrete neurologic evaluation (GCS scores) to twelve of the fourteen patients whose prolonged ICP problems required more aggressive management.

ICP and jugular venous monitoring was discontinued in most cases after 7 to 10 day because of resolution of increased ICP. During this interval six patients had SICH associated with prolonged hypoxic episodes, and six had SICH not associated with prolonged hypoxemia. The hypoxia-free group had no GCS decreases from their best GCS scores (range from 4 to 8), whereas all the patients with prolonged hypoxic episodes had GCS scores decreased to 3 and 4. While the two groups both had refractory ICP, they differed significantly with respect to changes in the GCS during the first week post injury ($p < .01$, paired t-test).

Outcome at 45 Days

One patient died early in his intensive care unit (ICU) treatment. Two additional patients died after the third postinjury week due to recurrent pneumonia and sepsis. Five patients were in the prolonged vegetative state category. Two of these five had GCS scores of 5 and 6 with negligible signs of recovery, while the remaining three had slowly regained some motor activity and had GCS scores of 8. Eight of the sixteen patients (50%) had recovered consciousness; however, six of these patients still were disoriented or had speech problems (GCS scores of 13 to 15).

Two of the eight patients who had regained consciousness at 45 day had sustained grade I or II hypoxemia and SICH, four others had SICH but no prolonged hypoxic events, and the other two had neither a prolonged hypoxic event nor SICH although both of them had had brief hypoxic episodes that quickly responded to treatment. Of the three patients who died, all had had prolonged hypoxic events unresponsive to treatment and SICH. The five patients in a prolonged vegetative state all had SICH. In addition, three had prolonged hypoxic events unresponsive to treatment, while two had SICH in the absence of prolonged hypoxic insults. One of these later patients was perplexing in that he had an increase in his GCS from 5 to 10 while being vigorously treated for SICH for 10 day but then had a gradual worsening of his neurologic status (GCS dropped to 8) in the absence of intracranial hypertension, inadequate systemic oxygenation, or hemodynamic instability (Figure 5.5).

DISCUSSION

Technical Standards

Monitoring cerebral oxygen extraction requires measurement of both the jugular venous and arterial oxygen content. It is difficult to identify acute hypoxemia and even more difficult to assess rapidly whether acute treatment for correcting the hypoxemia is sufficient. The indwelling oximeter catheter allows for increased sophistication of serial $AJDO_2$ measurements and substantially improves patient care by identifying sudden and significant SaO_2 drops and providing parameters by which interventions could be evaluated. Our data would indicate that hypoxic events are common and that those events that are prolonged—that is, not quickly remedial to treatment—are associated with a significant decrease in neurologic outcome.

The methodology has limitations. SjO_2 may be falsely high due to a leftward shift of the oxyhemoglobin dissociation curve as occurs with respiratory alkalosis. This might result in misleading information suggesting luxury perfusion when in fact the oxygen delivery may be compromised [23]. By measuring

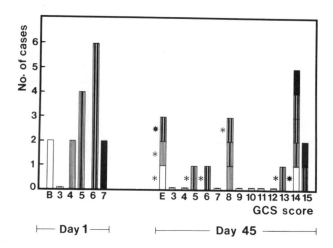

Figure 5.5 Distribution of GCS scores among the sixteen subjects at two stages after injury. On the right side is a brick-laying rearrangement of the new scores and the corresponding number of cases, matched with their initial graphic representation. B: scores not assessable due to barbiturate coma; E: patients who expired; open asterisk: patients who sustained prolonged hypoxemic insults at grades II and III; heavy circled asterisk: patients who sustained prolonged grade I hypoxemia.

oxygen tension intermittently and comparing it with the continuous oximeter values, we have found that SjO_2 closely parallels PjO_2 even during the extreme hypocapnia we utilized in many of these patients for ICP control.

Jugular venous measurements reflect global brain oxygen extraction and may not reflect regional metabolism. However, experience with regional CBF measurements and $AJDO_2$ clearly indicates that patients with predominantly diffuse CT findings have far more important global than regional flow changes, especially while being hyperventilated [19]. Indeed, if hyperventilation effectively minimizes the effects of heterogeneous perfusion on $AJDO_2$, it seems reasonable to accept oligemic SjO_2 values as indicative of a process with global consequences than as just a global measurement. Because we do support this notion, subjects were not included in this monitoring series if not requiring hyperventilation therapy for ICP control. Furthermore, it is difficult to believe that a global measurement that indicated hypoxemia does not reflect that a portion, and possibly a very large portion, of the brain is in fact hypoxemic. From the corollary, when the global measurement indicates hyperemia, it is not intuitively clear that the whole brain is hyperemic. However, regional CBF measurements do support the relationship between a narrow $AJDO_2$ and diffuse cerebral hyperemia. The final significant concern is that there is an immensely important part of the central nervous system that is not assessed by the jugular venous measurements. Clearly, in terms of relative tissue weight, the posterior fossa blood flow contributes insignificantly to the jugular bulb outflow, and thus, measurements of global oxygen extraction do not provide adequate information relative to brain stem and cerebellar blood flow. It is for these reasons that oxygen extraction monitoring must not be thought of as a replacement for critical, detailed, repetitive clinical evaluation. Indeed, two of these patients developed bilateral pupillary dilation in the absence of oligemic $AJDO_2$ values. In one case vasospasm of the posterior circulation was strongly suggested [20], while the other case raised the question of whether metabolism and blood flow matching is significantly affected by barbiturate intoxication.

We previously postulated that widened $AJDO_2$ values suggestive of global ischemia could be induced by standard hyperventilation therapy [4,11,19]. The most striking evidence of cerebral oligemia was provided by a case in whom cerebrovascular resistance gradually increased not only as a consequence of moderate hyperventilation but also by the development of a delayed intracerebral hematoma. Those events resulted in a relatively minor neurologic deterioration but a nearly twofold increase in $AJDO_2$. In a group of unparalyzed patients with predominantly diffuse brain CT findings, we were able to identify a rather peculiar neurologic pattern: normal brain stem reflexes, no pathologic posturing, steady deterioration to uni- or bilateral flexor and eventually extensor posturing, and $AJDO_2$ widening. Auditory brain stem evoked potentials were also repeatedly normal. These patients had well-controlled ICP and normal CPPs, and therefore, a correlation between continuous hyperventilation therapy, oligemia, and progressive neurologic deterioration was strongly indicated. These findings further enhanced the significance of $AJDO_2$ monitoring for global cerebral ischemia and provided the rationale for attempting to reverse increases in O_2 extraction.

In a different group of patients, evaluated by positron emission tomographic (PET) scanning, increased regional O_2 extraction fractions were found to correlate with neurologic signs due to ischemic infarction [21]. Should global cerebral oxygen extraction parameters deserve the same relevance, our methodology would be further supported.

Monitoring Hypoxemia

Continuous arterial oximetry was the most gratifying patient management technique in this system. The short response time, range alarms on the system, and excellent agreement with conventional oximetry made the femoral arterial catheter monitoring a most valuable management tool. Undoubtedly, the most surprising contribution of arterial oximetry monitoring was the ability to detect sudden SaO_2 decreases. Frequently these hypoxic events were not associated with a clearly recognized etiology, but they did occur. Indeed, the majority of the early hypoxic episodes promptly responded to increases in inspired oxygen concentration (FIO_2), but without this monitoring system they surely would have gone undetected until the patient deteriorated, the ICP rose, or other deleterious events occurred.

Our data indicate that prompt reversibility of acute hypoxemia in the early phase, when pulmonary complications are generally absent or minor, was accomplished in a nearly automatic manner by standard FIO_2 modulations, presumably avoiding prolonged hypoxemic episodes. In contrast, within a few days post injury, severe pulmonary complications were more frequent, occasionally associated with systemic hemodynamic instability, and frequently precluded a simple resolution of these hypoxic and ischemic insults. Thus, the duration of the hypoxemia was substantially longer than in the early stages after injury. Unfortunately, the occurrence of these prolonged hypoxemic insults significantly correlated with neurologic deterioration, during or even after periods of intracranial hypertension. However, at least we were able to define a cause for these otherwise unexplainable neurologic changes and to initiate prompt therapy. CT brain scans obtained in these patients after these events demonstrated residual brain swelling in five of six cases. These observations are in agreement with animal studies in which brain swelling complicated by hypoxemia yielded significantly more pronounced neurologic worsening than did brain swelling alone [14].

SUMMARY

Unequivocal evidence of the malignant repercussions of intractable intracranial hypertension is a common experience for those treating severely head-injured patients and is well documented in the literature [14,22–24]. Our experience demonstrates that secondary hypoxic cerebral insults are frequent and of clinical relevance even in patients whose mechanical ventilatory support appears satisfactory. Our monitoring scheme makes it possible for the multidisciplinary care team to intervene, on a more rational basis, for the patient's benefit prior to neurologic deterioration. This is the most powerful rationale for any monitoring system of cerebral physiology. We anticipate that constant monitoring of jugular venous oxygen will not be required since most changes in that system are relatively slow or predicted from changes in arterial blood pressure or oxygen tension. However, we do find that the supplemental monitoring system is valuable over prolonged periods of time to care for these desperately injured patients.

ACKNOWLEDGMENTS

The authors are greatly indebted to James W. Hall III, Ph.D., for the performance and interpretation of auditory brain stem evoked potentials; to Steven J. Allen, M.D., and other members of the Hermann Hospital Surgical ICU staff for significant contribution in patient management; and to Glenis M. Withell, R.N., for help in data analysis and preparation of the manuscript. This work was supported in part by NIH Grant Number N01-NS-9-2314B.

REFERENCES

1. Gibbs EL, Lennox WG, Nims LF, Gibbs FA. Arterial and cerebral venous blood. Arterial-venous differences in man. J Biol Chem 1942;144:325–32.
2. Kety SS, Schmidt CF. The nitrous oxide method for the quantitative determination of cerebral blood flow in man: theory, procedure, and normal values. J Clin Invest 1948;27:476–83.
3. Guillaume J, Janny P. Manometrie intracranienne continue: interet de la method et premiers resultats. Rev Neurol 1951;84:131–42.
4. Lundberg N. Continuous recording and control of ventricular fluid pressure in neurosurgical practice. Acta Psychiatr Neurol Scand 1960;36(Suppl. 149):1–193.
5. Langfitt TW, Weinstein JD, Kassell NF. Cerebral vasomotor paralysis produced by intracranial hypertension. Neurology 1965;15:622–41.
6. Langfitt TW, Weinstein JD, Sklar FH, Zaren HA, Kassell NF. Contribution of intracranial blood volume to three forms of experimental brain swelling. Johns Hopkins Med J 1968;122:261–70.
7. Bruce DA, Langfitt TW, Miller JD, Schultz H, Vapalahti M, Stanek A, Goldberg HI. Regional cerebral blood flow, intracranial pressure, and brain metabolism in comatose patients. J Neurosurg 1973;38:131–44.
8. Enevoldsen EM, Cold G, Jensen FT, Malmros R. Dynamic changes in regional CBF, intraventricular pressure, CSF pH and lactate levels during the acute phase of head injuries. J Neurosurg 1976;44:191–214.

9. Fieschi C, Battistini N, Beduschi A, Boselli L, Rossanda M. Regional cerebral blood flow and intraventricular pressure in acute head injuries. J Neurol Neurosurg Psychiat 1974;37:1378–88.

10. Obrist WD, Gennarelli TA, Segawa H, Dolinskas CA, Langfitt TW. Relation of cerebral blood flow to neurological status and outcome in head-injured patients. J Neurosurg 1979;51:292–300.

11. Obrist WD, Cruz J, Jaggi JL, Langfitt TW. CBF and intracranial hypertension in acute head injury. J Cer Blood Flow Metab 1983;3(Suppl 1):S67–68.

12. Overgaard J, Tweed WA. Cerebral circulation after head injury. Part 1: cerebral blood flow and its regulation after closed head injury with emphasis on clinical correlations. J Neurosurg 1974;41:531–41.

13. Overgaard J, Mosdal C, Tweed WA. Cerebral circulation after head injury. Part 3: does reduced regional cerebral blood flow determine recovery of brain function after blunt head injury? J Neurosurg 1981;55:63–74.

14. Grubb RL, Jr., Raichle ME, Phelps ME, Ratcheson RA. Effects of increased intracranial pressure on cerebral blood volume, blood flow, and oxygen utilization in monkeys. J Neurosurg 1975;43:385–98.

15. Cold GE. Cerebral metabolic rate of oxygen ($CMRO_2$) in the acute phase of brain injury. Acta Anaesth Scand 1978;22:249–56.

16. Finnerty AF, Witkin L, Fazekas JF. Cerebral hemodynamics during cerebral ischemia induced by acute hypotension. J Clin Invest 1954;33:1227–32.

17. Kety SS, King BD, Horvath SM, Jeffers WA, Hafkenschiel JH. The effects of an acute reduction in blood pressure by means of differential spinal sympathetic block on the cerebral circulation of hypertensive patients. J Clin Invest 1950;29:402–07.

18. Gotoh F, Meyer JS, Takagi Y. Cerebral effects of hyperventilation in man. Arch Neurol 1965;12:410–23.

19. Obrist WD, Langfitt TW, Jaggi JL, Cruz J, Gennarelli TA. Cerebral blood flow and metabolism in comatose patients with acute head injury: relationship to intracranial hypertension. J Neurosurg 1984;61:241–53.

20. Cruz J, Langfitt TW, Obrist WD. Detection of brain ischemia in head injured patients by measurement of serial arteriojugular O_2 differences. Presented at the Annual Meeting of the American Association of Neurological Surgeons, San Francisco, California, April 8–12, 1984.

21. Baele PL, McMichan JC, Marsh HM, Sill C, Southorn PA. Continuous monitoring of mixed venous oxygen saturation in critically ill patients. Anesth Analg 1982;61:513–17.

22. Cruz J, Miner ME, Allen SJ. Modulating cerebral oxygen delivery in coma following acute diffuse brain injury. Soc Neurosci Abstr 1984;10:542.

23. Larson CP, Jr., Ehrenfeld WK, Wade JG, Wylie E. Jugular venous oxygen saturation as an index of adequacy of cerebral oxygenation. Surgery 1967;62:31–39.

24. Marshall LF, Bruce DA, Bruno L, Langfitt TW. Vertebrobasilar spasm: a significant cause of neurological deficit in head injury. J Neurosurg 1978;48:560–64.

Chapter 6

The Metabolic Response to Severe Head Injury

Guy L. Clifton
Claudia S. Robertson

A similarity between the autonomic status of patients with severe head injury and those with burns of the body surface has been observed. Both demonstrate hypertension, tachycardia, hyperthermia, and wasting of body mass with seemingly adequate nutrition [1–4]. The work of Wilmore and others has shown a relationship between the intensity of the hypermctabolic state of burned patients and a hyperadrenergic state as reflected by increased urinary epinephrine and norepinephrine [5]. Two manifestations of a hyperadrenergic state in patients with burns, sepsis, and systemic trauma are increased nutritional requirements or hypermetabolism and a hyperdynamic cardiovascular state in which there is an increased delivery of oxygen to the tissues. Both have implications for management of the patient with a systemic insult and may, therefore, be important in head injury management. The hyperdynamic cardiovascular state has been associated with an increased need for intravascular volume to sustain increased oxygen delivery in burned patients and postresuscitated shock patients [6,7]. Nutritional management of hypermetabolism is believed to be a major factor in the outcome of head-injured and burned patients [8,9]. Both a hyperdynamic cardiovascular state and a hypermetabolic nutritional state have been shown in head-injured patients [3,4,10].

The purposes of this study, relative to the hyperdynamic cardiovascular state, were to provide further understanding of the relationship between the hyperadrenergic state, the severity of neurologic injury, and the intensity of the hyperdynamic cardiovascular response. All patients were maintained with a pulmonary capillary wedge pressure (PCWP) of ≥ 8 mm Hg, thus avoiding dehydration. Normal or increased plasma volume was required to maintain optimal cardiac function as judged by PCWP and cardiac output, and an important management question was whether failure to fluid restrict patients resulted in an increased incidence of increased intracranial pressure (ICP) in a consecutive series of patients.

The purposes of this study relative to the hypermetabolic nutritional

73

response in head injury were to determine the relationship between the level of caloric consumption and two factors that could potentially have the greatest influence upon it: temperature and Glasgow Coma Scale (GCS) score. A management question to be answered was the extent to which enteral alimentation is capable of meeting the caloric requirements of head-injured patients in the acute phase of head injury.

METHODS

Patient Population and Selection

The patients studied came from a group of 122 patients in coma from all causes including patients sustaining gunshot wounds to the brain with a GCS score of ≤ 7 for at least 6 hr after admission or who deteriorated to coma after head injury. Patients who met brain death criteria on admission were excluded from study. The following data were prospectively recorded for the 2 yr period of study for all patients in coma for 6 hr or longer after head injury: initial GCS, duration of coma, time of death, pathologic diagnosis, outcome at 3 mo, and demographic characteristics such as age and sex. Table 6.1 gives the age distribution, sex, initial GCS, primary diagnosis, clinical course, and outcome at 3 mo of all patients in coma from head injury for the 2 yr period of study. The characteristics of 55 patients who underwent cardiovascular and metabolic study are compared with the consecutive series of 122 patients.

The selection of patients for detailed physiologic study was random with one exception. It can be seen that patients with a brief duration of coma (less than 48 hr) are underrepresented in the physiologic studies. These patients often rapidly awoke after removal of an extracerebral hematoma or had a normal computerized tomography (CT) scan and rapidly awoke. Since their central nervous system (CNS) injury was often mild, it was not possible or necessary to monitor cardiovascular and metabolic parameters in many of these patients. Otherwise, the groups undergoing physiologic study are representative and make up 57% of the total population of patients who were in coma more than 48 hr.

Patient Management

Mean time from injury to hospital admission was 2 hr. Patients were intubated in the emergency department, and mannitol 1 gm/kg, phenytoin 18 mg/kg, and dexamethasone 10 to 25 mg were given intravenously. CT scans were performed after initial management. Only 5% of patients had associated injuries requiring laparotomy or thoracotomy. Hematomas were removed immediately after recognition on CT scan. An ICP monitor, either a ventriculostomy (80%) or a subarachnoid bolt, was placed in the operating room in all patients. In the

Table 6.1 Demographic and Clinical Characteristics of Consecutive Series and of Study Group

Demographics	Cardiovascular Study Only	Metabolic Study Only	Both Studies	No Physio-logic Studies	Total Series
Number	20	11	24	67	122
Age					
15 to 20 yr	3	0	3	9	15
21 to 30 yr	10	5	12	36	63
31 to 40 yr	2	1	5	8	16
41 to 50 yr	3	3	1	5	12
> 50	2	2	3	9	16
Sex					
Male	17	11	21	62	111
Female	3	0	3	5	11
Initial GCS					
3	0	0	0	6	6
4 to 5	9	4	7	24	44
6 to 7	11	7	17	37	72
Duration of coma					
< 48 hr	2	2	2	30	36
48 hr to 7 day	5	4	9	25	43
> 7 day	13	5	13	12	43

Table 6.1 (Continued)

Demographics	Cardiovascular Study Only	Metabolic Study Only	Both Studies	No Physiologic Studies	Total Series
Pathologic diagnosis					
EDH = epidural hematoma	3	0	0	11	14
SDH = subdural hematoma	3	2	2	14	21
ICH = intracerebral hematoma	3	5	7	7	22
DBI = diffuse brain injury	10	1	8	23	42
GSW = gunshot wound	1	3	7	12	23
Outcome at 3 mo					
GR = good recovery	5	3	9	21	38
MD = moderate disability	4	2	6	7	19
SD = severe disability	1	3	3	4	11
PVS = persistent vegetative state	1	3	6	4	14
Died	9	0	0	31	40

operating room or on admission to the intensive care unit, a radial arterial cathether and Swan-Ganz catheter were placed. Swan-Ganz catheters and radial arterial cathethers were changed or removed after 72 hr and ICP monitors were removed after 72 hr if ICP remained below 20 mm Hg. Swan-Ganz catheters were used for more prolonged periods in patients who had systemic hypertension or intracranial hypertension.

Management in the intensive care unit was by protocol. Patients were routinely hyperventilated with head elevation. Fluid restriction was not used, and PCWP was kept $\geq$ 8 mm Hg. Morphine and pancuronium bromide were used first if ICP rose, then ventricular drainage followed by mannitol. Dehydration was prevented during mannitol administration by replacement of urinary fluid losses. The routine use of morphine was minimized because of its tendency to produce intolerance of feedings.

Two protocols were used in managing the thirty-five patients who underwent detailed nutritional study. In the first fifteen patients enteral alimentation with a formula containing 2 kcal/cc and 14% of calories from protein (Magnacal, Organon) was used with advancement to a maximum rate of 100 cc/hr as rapidly as tolerated. Enteral feedings were begun at 50 cc/hr by continuous infusion and increased by 20 cc every 12 hr to a maximum rate of 100 cc/hr. Feedings were decreased for a gastric residual volume of $\geq$300 cc measured every 4 hr. In the fifteen patients studied with this protocol, resting metabolic expenditure (RME) was measured daily for the first 9 day. In the other twenty patients a study was conducted comparing the effectiveness at isocaloric feeding of two different formulas in achieving nitrogen equilibrium, one formula containing 22% protein calories and 1.5 kcal/cc (Traumacal, Mead Johnson), and the other, 14% protein calories and 2 kcal/cc (Magnacal, Organon). In the second protocol RME measurement was carried out at 3 to 5 day intervals, and feedings advanced as rapidly as possible untidl 150% of measured RME was being replaced by enteral feeding. RME measurements were performed in both protocols during maximal enteral feeding with formulas containing caloric densities of 1.5 to 2 kcal/cc.

Cardiovascular Methods

A total of 265 cardiovascular measurements were made one to three times daily during the first 3 day after injury. Sampling was begun within 24 hr of admission for all patients but not within 12 hr of anesthetic administration or volume expansion. The thermodilution technique of measuring cardiac output was used. Plasma volume was measured by an isotope dilution technique using radioiodinated serum albumin. Mean PCWP during sampling was 8 to 12 mm Hg. When necessary, morphine and pancuronium bromide were used to stop spontaneous movement. Some cardiovascular samples were taken during spontaneous posturing and after administration of antihypertensive drugs, but these data were analyzed separately. Samples included in this chapter are from patients without elevated ICP at the time of sampling. The following parameters were recorded at each sampling: mean arterial pressure (MAP), pulmonary artery pressure (PAP), pulmonary capillary wedge pressure (PCWP), heart rate (HR), temperature (T), ICP, central venous pressure (CVP), mixed venous and arterial blood gases, plasma epinephrine and norepinephrine, hemoglobin, and GCS. Parameters calculated from these directly measured values were arteriovenous oxygen differences ($AVDO_2$), oxygen consumption (VO_2), oxygen availability (O_2Av), cardiac index (CI), stroke index (SI), systemic vascular resistance (SVR), pulmonary vascular resistance (PVR), left and right cardiac work (LCW and RCW), left and right ventricular stroke work (LVSW and RVSW), and pulmonary venous admixture (QS/QT).

Arterial epinephrine and norepinephrine were measured in plasma taken from the arterial catheter and the Swan-Ganz catheter just prior to each cardiovascular sampling. Samples of blood for epinephrine and norepinephrine were collected in a chilled solution of EGTA and glutathione 60 mg/ml and 90 mg/ml, respectively, immediately placed on ice at the bedside, and centrifuged. The supernatant was frozen at -20°C until samples were analyzed. The technique used is a modification of that described by Peuler and Johnson and uses catechol-o-methyl-transferase to convert epinephrine to ^3H metanephrine and norepinephrine to ^3H normetanephrine in the presence of ^3H methyl-s-adenosylmethionine as the methyl group donor [11]. The O-methylated metabolites of catechols were isolated by solvent extraction, separated by thin layer chromatography, and counted in a liquid scintillation counter.

Metabolic Methods

Caloric consumption was measured by indirect calorimetry using a Beckman MMC Horizon. A major potential source of error was lack of steady-state conditions. To ensure steady-state conditions, patients were not suctioned, turned, or stimulated for 15 min prior to sampling or during sampling. Patients were not studied when there had been any recent change in respiratory status or during spontaneous posturing. Heart rate, rectal temperature, and blood pressure were recorded at the time of sampling. Sampling times were from 20 min to 2 hr.

RESULTS

Cardiovascular Results

Cardiovascular measurements were performed during days 1 to 5 after injury for forty-four patients. Although most patients were comatose on admission to the hospital, three with diffuse brain injury were initially awake but then deteriorated after 2 to 5 day. For purposes of these analyses, day 1 in these three patients will be considered the day that they deteriorated rather than the first day after injury. The distribution of the type of injury, initial GCS, and outcome are shown in Table 6.1. The mean age of the group was 30 ± 11 yr, and no patient had any significant medical illnesses prior to the injury. From these forty-four patients, 265 sets of cardiovascular data were obtained. Data obtained while patients were in barbiturate coma, after patients became clinically brain dead, or during periods of elevated ICP (Cushing response) have been omitted, leaving 245 sets of data for subsequent analyses.

Description of the cardiovascular response (Table 6.2) lists the mean values of all variables measured and demonstrates the hyperdynamic cardiovascular pattern that occurred after head trauma. Resting metabolic requirements in the acute phase of injury were moderately elevated. The mean VO_2 of the forty-four patients, here calculated by the Fick principle, were 159 ± 52 ml/min M^2, or about 14% greater than normal. Twenty-two patients had an average VO_2 greater than 140 ml/min M^2, and eleven had an average VO_2 greater than 165 ml/min M^2 during the first 5 day. These findings are similar to those obtained with indirect calorimetry. The main difference in the two methods is that indirect calorimetry reflects the average VO_2 over about 30 min, while the VO_2 calculated from $AVDO_2$ and CI is a more instantaneous value.

The most consistent hemodynamic finding after trauma was an elevated cardiac output. Thirty-nine of the forty-four patients studied had at least one increased cardiac output during the first 5 day. The mean CI of thirty-three patients was greater than 3.4 l/min/M^2, and the mean CI of fifteen patients was greater than 4.4 l/min/M^2. The patients who had the highest VO_2 typically had the highest CI. There was a linear relationship between VO_2 and CI ($n = 37$, $r = .57$, $p < .01$), suggesting that the increased cardiac output was in part a response to the elevated metabolic requirements.

Hypertension was the next most common hemodynamic finding in these head-injured patients. Thirty-four of the patients had at least one systolic BP greater than 160 mm Hg at the times of the cardiovascular studies. The hypertension often was transient or related to posturing and was treated simply by sedating or paralyzing the patient. Ten of the patients, however, had persistently elevated BP unrelated to increased ICP, requiring treatment with propranolol, supplemented by hydralazine or alpha methyldopa. Despite treatment, seven patients had an average systolic BP greater than 160 mm Hg. The hypertension associated with head trauma was predominantly a systolic hypertension and was different from essential hypertension, in which cardiac output is usually normal and SVR increased. Instead, the increased BP was a part of the hyperdynamic state and was dependent on increased HR ($n = 243$, $r = .17$, $p < .01$) and CI and not changes in SVR. The BP was also extremely labile and responded to external stimuli with an exaggerated increase. Twenty of the patients had an SVR less than 1,900 dynes sec/cm^5/M^2. Because of this vasodilation, plasma volume was greater than normal in twelve of twenty-two patients studied. Plasma volume data are summarized in Table 6.3.

Table 6.2 Mean Metabolic and Cardiopulmonary Values in Forty-four Comatose Patients during Days 1 to 5 after Injury

		Units	Normal Values	Head-injured Patient Values
Metabolic	RME (Indirect calorimetry)	kcal/24 hr	Varies with sex, BSA	2459 ± 533
	VO$_2$ (oxygen consumption, Fick principle)	ml/min × M^2	140 ± 25	259 ± 52
Cardiac	HR (heart rate)	beats/min	71 ± 4	83 ± 15
	Preload			
	CVP (central venous pressure)	mm Hg	5 ± 2	9 ± 4
	PCWP (pulmonary capillary wedge pressure)	mm Hg	8 ± 3	11 ± 4
	LVEDV (left ventricular end diastolic volume)	ml/M^2	70 ± 20	106 ± 34
	Afterload			
	MAP (mean arterial pressure)	mm Hg	90 ± 5	105 ± 7
	SVR (systemic vascular resistance)	dynes × sec/cm^5 × M^2	2180 ± 210	1998 ± 443
	Performance			
	CI (cardiac index)	l/min × M^2	3.2 ± 0.2	4.2 ± 0.9
	SI (stroke index)	ml/beat × M^2	46 ± 5	50 ± 9
	LVSW (left ventricular stroke work)	gm-M/M^2	56 ± 6	73 ± 14
Pulmonary	PVR (pulmonary vascular resistance)	dynes × sec/cm^5 × M^2	270 ± 45	112 ± 58
	QS/QT (pulmonary venous admixture)	%	6 ± 2	14 ± 5

*Relationship of GCS, VO₂, and Cardiovascular Variables
to Plasma Catecholamines*

To investigate the relationship between sympathetic hyperactivity and the cardiovascular response, twenty of the patients had a total of ninety-eight measurements of arterial epinephrine and norepinephrine at the times of their cardiovascular measurements. The mean value of norepinephrine for ten patients on day 1 with a GCS of 4 to 5 was 890 ± 508 pg/ml, and for patients with a GCS of 6 to 7, it was 431 ± 165 pg/ml. The mean values were significantly different ($p<.05$). Epinephrine was also significantly higher in posturing patients than in localizing patients. Mean epinephrine for posturing patients was 214 ± 172 pg/ml and that for patients with GCS of 6 to 7 was 63 ± 32 pg/ml. Normal values for epinephrine and norepinephrine are 0 to 55 pg/ml and 65 to 320 pg/ml respectively.

MAP measured on day 1 in forty-four patients was not different between patients with a GCS of 4 to 5 and 6 to 7 (GCS 4 to 5, 105 ± 6 mm Hg; GCS 6 to 7, 105 ± 18 mm Hg). CI on day 1 was significantly higher in those with a posturing response (4.5 ± 0.9 l/min x M²) than in those with a localizing motor response (3.8 l/min x M²). The elevation of CI in patients with a posturing motor response was associated with an increased VO_2. The mean VO_2 for patients with GCS 4 to 5 was 177 ± 64 ml/min x M² and that for localizing patients was 143 ± 33 ml/min/M².

VO_2 was related to both arterial epinephrine ($n=78$, $r=.50$, $p<.01$) and arterial norepinephrine ($n=78$, $r=.30$, $p<.01$). Many of the other cardiovascular variables were also correlated with catecholamines when tested by regression analysis by the method of least squares. Arterial epinephrine was related to MAP ($n=89$, $r=.41$, $p<.01$), CI ($n=89$, $r=.21$, $p<.05$), HR ($n=88$, $r=.46$, $p<.01$), LCW ($n=88$, $r=.33$, $p<.01$, $AVDO_2$ ($n=78$, $r=.33$, $p<.01$), but not SI, SVR, LVSW, PVR, or RVSW. Arterial norepinephrine was related to MAP ($n=89$, $r=.38$, $p<.01$), CI ($n=89$, $r=.22$, $p<.05$), SI ($n=88$, $r=.23$, $p<.05$), HR ($n=88$, $r=.50$, $p<.01$), LCW ($n=88$, $r=.32$, $p<.01$), RVSW ($n=85$, $r=.24$, $p<.05$), $r=.21$, $p<.05$) but not SVR, LVSW, PVR, or $AVDO_2$.

Effect of Normovolemia on ICP

Table 6.3 illustrates the plasma volume measurements made during the first 3 day after injury for twenty-two patients. The mean values are slightly elevated. Intake and output records for these patients are also shown and illustrate approximately 3,500 cc/24 hr of fluid replacement and urinary loss.

Table 6.4 shows the general characteristics of this series and other published series with similar management protocols though not specifically emphasizing normovolemia and early nutrition. Only data from ninety-nine patients with nonpenetrating injuries from this series are shown for purposes of comparison of ICP incidence. The series are similar in average age and percentage of posturing patients. This series differs most significantly in a higher

Table 6.3 Plasma Volume and PCWP in the First 3 Days after Injury for Twenty-two Patients

Intravascular Volume	Day 1	Day 2	Day 3
Mean plasma volume (Normal = 960 − 1,560 ml/M²)	1,622 ± 204	1,692 ± 300	1,748 ± 326
Mean PCWP, mm Hg	10 ± 5	12 ± 6	11 ± 5
Fluid balance			
Intake/24 hr, ml	3,162 ± 1,018	3,889 ± 857	3,746 ± 935
Output/24 hr, ml	3,213 ± 1,753	3,668 ± 1,336	3,504 ± 1,034

Table 6.4 Comparison of Head Injury Series

Characteristic	Houston	Richmond	San Diego	Baltimore
Number	99	148	100	106
Average age, yr	32	27	32	29
Mass lesions, % of total	58%	40%	25%	31%
Decorticate, decerebrate, flaccid, % of total	39%	46%	45%	42%
Good recovery/moderate disability (3 mo), % of total	50%	60%	60%	50%
Incidence of ICP, >15 to 25 mm Hg	31% (20 mm Hg)	40% (20 mm Hg)	55% (15 mm Hg)	25% (25 mm Hg)
Death from uncontrolled ICP (Map = ICP), % of total	14%	14%	8%	14%
All deaths from neurologic causes, % of total	18%	14%	8%	14%
Deaths from systemic causes, % of total	7%	16%	20%	14%
Associated injury, % of total	2%	—	—	7%
Sepsis, % of total	5%	—	—	7%
Series mortality rate, % of total	25%	30%	28%	28%

percentage of patients with hematomas, reflecting a preponderance of injuries from assaults and falls. Fifty percent good recovery/moderate disability are seen in the Houston and Baltimore series and 60% in those from Richmond and San Diego [12–15]. The incidence of increased ICP varies with the level of elevation used for definition of increased ICP but is similar in this series to others (31%). The incidence of death from uncontrolled ICP in this series is 14% and very similar to other reported figures. About half the number of systemic deaths are found in this series than in others, but this figure is offset by a slight increase in the number of neurologic deaths not related to increased ICP, so that overall case mortality within all four series is similar though slightly lower in this series than in others. It may be concluded that normo-volemia has not produced an increased incidence of elevated ICP and may have been associated with a reduction in deaths from systemic causes.

Metabolic Results

Metabolic Characteristics

VO_2 and caloric expenditure were measured by indirect calorimetry 202 times in thirty-five patients. Four hundred sixteen days of nitrogen balance were obtained in thirty-four patients. RMEs of comatose patients following head injury were moderately elevated, an average of 50% greater than expected for patients of the same sex, age, and body size. Severity of neurologic injury was the major determinant of caloric requirements. Patients with posturing responses had a significantly higher RME than patients who withdrew or localized to painful stimuli; $168 \pm 53\%$ and $129 \pm 31\%$ of expected respectively. There was no difference in the mean percentage of RME replaced or in mean temperature in the two groups of patients.

At a given severity of neurologic injury, temperature affected RME. Temperatures were plotted against RME for all days of study for patients with a GCS of 6 to 7 and of 4 to 5 and analyzed by regression analysis. Body temperature increased RME by 45% of expected per °C in patients with a GCS of 4 to 5 ($n = 23$, $r = .63$, $p < .01$) and by 15% of expected per °C in patients with a GCS of 6 to 7 ($n = 49$, $r = .37$, $p < .01$). There was no consistent change in RME with temperature in patients with a GCS greater than 8. Patients with RME measurement and GCS ≥ 8 were those who had neurologically improved from a comatose state, and RME was probably influenced by many other variables such as activity, pain, and muscle tone in these patients. Arterial catecholamines obtained during fifty-nine determinations of RME by indirect calorimetry did not show a significant relationship to the RME probably because of the rapidly changing nature of plasma epinephrine and norepinephrine and the long collection period of indirect calorimetry.

Ability of Enteral Alimentation to Meet Caloric Requirements

Table 6.5 shows the balance periods of study with measured RME and average percentage of RME replaced during the balance period of thirty-five patients. The mean time from injury to the beginning of enteral feedings for the thirty-five patients who underwent metabolic study was 1 day. Two study patients

Table 6.5 Balance Period of Maximal Enteral Intake for
Thirty-five Patients

GCS at Start of Balance Period	Average RME of Balance Period (Percent Expected)	Days after Injury of Balance Period	Mean Percent RME Replaced
6	156	1 to 7	166
4	119	1 to 26	131
4	180	4 to 9	166
7	109	1 to 5	113
5	140	16 to 13	196
8	99.6	4 to 9	138
4	155	18 to 21	101
8	131	1 to 5	150
6	149	2 to 6	91
7	138	2 to 7	135
7	119	1 to 6	168
4	144	1 to 10	103
8	123	2 to 5	190
7	74	1 to 9	200
	(Barbiturate coma)		
10	143	9 to 5	135
7	136	4 to 10	145
7	131	4 to 10	143
10	147	2 to 8	132
10	119	7 to 13	149
6	188	12 to 18	145
10	186	3 to 9	127
10	138	14 to 20	144
10	167	13 to 19	146
8	168	2 to 8	123
10	135	14 to 20	136
10	196	12 to 18	127
11	114	4 to 10	149
5	114	2 to 8	149
7	121	4 to 10	145
6	143	3 to 9	176
6	145	8 to 14	129
10	188	16 to 22	125
11	176	6 to 12	127
6	132	7 to 12	142
10	122	15 to 19	160

did not tolerate enteral feeding until the eighth postinjury day, and one of
these received intravenous hyperalimentation. The mean time from injury to
100% RME replacement was 3 day. For each patient enteral feedings were
escalated to either 150% of RME or a rate of 100 cc/hr of formula and

maintained at that level. The mean time from injury to maximal alimentation was 6 day. While replacement of 100% RME occurred within a few days after injury for most patients, nitrogen intakes of > 15 gm were not achieved until an average of 6 day postinjury with wide variations among patients in the time that they tolerated maximal alimentation. Although caloric requirements were readily met, net nitrogen equilibrium was attained in only seven patients and then only when greater than 125% of RME was replaced at levels of nitrogen inttake of 20 to 35 gm/24 hr. The limiting factor in enteral alimentation was gastric tolerance of feedings.

DISCUSSION

Several questions important to head injury management are raised by the finding of a hypermetabolic state in head-injured patients and by the management principles that are evolving in treatment of this response in burned and multiply injured patients. Maintenance of normal or elevated plasma volume as guided by a normal PCWP has not been found in this study to predispose to brain swelling and may help to diminish fatal systemic complications of fluid restriction such as renal failure from dehydration. The effect of dehydration on oxygen delivery to the brain is another major concern. With the very large urine outputs documented in these patients and the dependence of cardiac function in some patients on a high preload, a program of fluid restriction could well result in a fall in cardiac output, a fall in cerebral blood flow, and resulting cerebral ischemia. The more severe the neurologic injury, the more intense the hyperadrenergic and hypermetabolic states become. In some patients the maintenance of normovolemia may be of particular importance. In management of the multiply traumatized patient with a head injury, volume depletion could impair supply of oxygen and glucose to damaged organs and increase mortality rate. A situation where hypermetabolism is met by inadequate oxygen delivery is destructive. Monitoring of jugular venous oxygen content is a simple and effective way of detecting this situation in head-injured patients and a useful guide to the effects of systemic therapy on cerebral circulation and metabolism.

Another important management aspect of the hypermetabolic response is nutrition. These studies have shown that enteral alimentation may be administered and is tolerated within the first few days of injury in most severely head-injured patients. With slow progression of feeding to provide 100% of RME within 4 day of injury, intolerance of feedings and diarrhea were seldom a problem. One hundred fifty percent replacement of measured RME was achieved on the average by the eighth post-injury day in twenty consecutive patients, but nitrogen equilibrium was not achieved unless well in excess of 150% RME was replaced. Maintaining this level of calorie intake for a sustained period of time was possible. Based on data obtained during periods of low intake, it can be concluded that the sedated patient with a posturing response to pain may have an RME of 70% over normal lasting at least for 20 day after injury. The localizing patient may have an RME of 30% over normal. Temperature may result in a marked increase in caloric requirements in the posturing patient (45%/°C). These values provide a reasonable index to nutritional replacement whether enteral or parenteral therapy is used.

The major research question raised by this study is what is the optimal physiologic milieu for recovery of the brain? At present, half of head injury mortalities result from uncontrolled ICP. With use of barbiturate coma, this percentage may be reduced. The neurologic outcome and ultimate mortality rate, even with an ability to control ICP in all patients, remains an important and unanswered question. Fifty percent of head injury deaths have been the result of systemic complications. How many of these are early complications in patients with recoverable injuries is unknown. Improved systemic management might result in fewer mortalities of patients with recoverable injuries. The relative constancy of the head injury mortality rate among current series of intensively managed patients would suggest that we may be approaching an irreducible head injury mortality rate determined by the severity of the initial injury. It may also suggest that some effort should center on achieving improved neurologic recovery in the 70 to 75% of patients who can be expected to survive with current management techniques by seeking the answers to questions such as the protein and amino acid needs of the acutely injured brain and how cardiac function and plasma volume relate to cerebral blood flow.

REFERENCES

1. Aulic LM, Wilmore DW, Goodwin CW, Becker RA. Increased visceral blood flow in burn patients. Fed Proc 1979;38:902.
2. Aulic LM, Wilmore DW, Mason AD, Jr, Pruitt BA, Jr. Influence of the burn wound on peripheral circulation in thermally injured patients. Am J Physiol 1977;233:H520.
3. Clifton GL, Robertson CS, Kyper K, Taylor A, Dhekne R, Grossman RG. Cardiovascular response to severe head injury. J Neurosurg 1983;59:447.
4. Schulte am Esch J, Murday H, Pfeifer G. Hemodynamic changes in patients with severe head injury. Acta Neurochir 1980;54:243.
5. Wilmore DW, Long JM, Mason AD, Jr, Skreen RW, Pruitt BA. Catecholamines: mediator of the hypermetabolic response to thermal injury. Ann Surg 1974;180:653.
6. Shoemaker WC, Appel PL, Waxman K, Schwartz S, Chang P. Clinical trial of survivors cardiorespiratory patterns as therapeutic goals in critically ill postoperative patients. Crit Care Med 1982; 10:398.
7. Shoemaker WC, Elwyn DH, Levin H, Rosen AL. Early prediction of death and survival in postoperative patients with circulatory shock by nonparametric analysis of cardiorespiratory variables. Crit Care Med 1974;2:317.
8. Alexander JW, MacMillan BG, Stinnett JE, Ogle C, Bozian RC, Fischer JE, Oakes JB, Morris MJ, Krummel R. Beneficial effects of aggressive protein feeding in severely burned children. Ann Surg 1980;192:505.
9. Rapp RP, Young B, Twyman D, Bivins BA, Haack D, Tibbs PA, Bean JR. The

favorable effect of early parenteral feeding on survival in head-injured patients. J Neurosurg 1983;58:906.

10. Clifton GL, Robertson CS, Grossman RG, Hodge S, Foltz R, Garza C. The metabolic response to severe head injury. J Neurosurg 1983;60:687.

11. Peuler JD, Johnson GA. Simultaneous single isotope radioenzymatic assay of plasma norepinephrine, epinephrine and dopamine. Life Sci 1977;21:625.

12. Becker DP, Miller JD, Ward JD, Greenberg RP, Young HF, Sakalas R. The outcome from severe head injury with early diagnosis and intensive management. J Neurosurg 1977;47:491.

13. Marshall LF, Smith RW, Shapiro HM. The outcome with aggressive treatment in severe head injuries. Part 1: the significance of intracranial pressure monitoring. J Neurosurg 1979;50:10.

14. Saul TG, Ducker TB. Effect of intracranial pressure monitoring and aggressive treatment on mortality in severe head injury. J Neurosurg 1982;56:498.

15. Robertson CS, Clifton GL, Grossman RG. Oxygen utilization and cardiovascular function in head-injured patients. Neurosurgery 1984;15:307.

Chapter 7

The Relative Durations of Coma and Posttraumatic Amnesia after Severe Nonmissile Head Injury: Findings from the Pilot Phase of the National Traumatic Coma Data Bank

Harvey S. Levin
Howard M. Eisenberg

Since Teasdale and Jennett developed the Glasgow Coma Scale (GCS), neurosurgeons have widely adopted this measure to assess the acute impairment of consciousness and duration of coma after head injury [1]. This advance in the assessment of impaired consciousness has permitted direct measurement of coma apart from the transitional, postcomatose stage of disturbed consciousness characterized by confusion, disorientation, and anterograde and retrograde amnesia. Although Russell [2] included both the periods of coma and subacute amnesia in his retrospective estimate of posttraumatic amnesia (PTA), newer investigations of the postcomatose period have directly monitored resolution of confusion, disorientation, and amnesia and redefined this interval as PTA [3,4].

From a clinical perspective, it would be useful to predict the duration of PTA given the duration of coma. Although this relationship has not been

We acknowledge the data contributed by Dr. Donald P. Becker, Medical College of Virginia; Dr. Robert G. Grossman, Baylor College of Medicine; Dr. John A. Jane, University of Virginia; Dr. Lawrence F. Marshall, University of California at San Diego; Dr. Kamran Tabaddor, Albert Einstein College of Medicine; and the assistance of Dr. Selma Kunitz, Office of Biometry and Field Studies, National Institute of Neurological and Communicative Disorders and Stroke.

specifically investigated, Jennett and Teasdale state that "an approximate guide to the relationship between return of speech and the end of PTA is that the interval from injury to the end of PTA is about four times longer than the interval until the patient first speaks (unless there has been a specific factor delaying the return of speech)" (p. 90) [5]. Although cases of severe, persistent anterograde amnesia (prolonged PTA) after relatively brief durations of coma or no loss of consciousness have been documented [6], no investigation has focused on the relative length of these intervals. Consequently, examination of the degree of relationship between the durations of coma and PTA is called for.

The effects of the type and lateralization of brain lesions on the duration of disturbed consciousness in head-injured patients also remain unclear. We compared the durations of coma and PTA in patients with severe head injury in whom we distinguished the presence of an intracranial mass lesion from a diffuse injury. Previous evidence has linked impairment of consciousness with insult to the language-dominant hemisphere in patients with acute cerebral infarction [7] and epileptics undergoing intracarotid sodium amytal injection [8]. Consequently, we compared the durations of coma and PTA in head-injured patients with left hemisphere mass lesions to the findings in cases with right hemisphere injury.

MATERIALS AND METHODS

Data from 50 right-handed survivors of nonmissile head injury were selected from the total series of 581 cases entered in the 3 yr pilot phase of the National Traumatic Coma Data Bank [9]. All patients had injuries that produced an initial GCS score of <8 following nonsurgical resuscitation or deterioration to a score of 8 or less during the first 48 hr after injury. The GCS was recorded every 8 hr during the patient's intensive care. The initial GCS score was 3 to 5 in 22 patients and 6 to 8 in 28 patients. Limitations on the sample size resulted from mortality and a delay in introducing a test to monitor PTA directly until the second year of the 3 yr pilot phase [4].

We defined the duration of coma exhaustively as the interval from the time of injury until the patient first exhibited eye opening to stimulation (E > 1), obeyed simple commands (M = 6), and uttered comprehensible words (V > 3). Cases who satisfied the first two criteria but who could not speak because of intubation or tracheostomy were also considered to be out of coma. Patients entered in the data bank who had complications precluding serial ratings of eye opening (e.g., ocular swelling) or motor response were excluded from this study. The duration of PTA was defined as the interval beginning with the termination of coma and ending when the Galveston Orientation and Amnesia Test (GOAT) score [4] improved to within normal limits (>75 on a 100 point scale). This definition of PTA duration, which is distinct from coma, yields a measure that has high interrater reliability [4]. We recognize that this direct, serial measurement differs from Russell's restropective method of estimating the total duration of disturbed consciousness—i.e., the combined durations of coma and failure to consolidate information about ongoing events [2].

The distinction drawn between diffuse injury and injury with mass lesion (Table 7.1) was based on a computed tomography (CT) scan obtained within 24 hr of injury and surgical findings. We classified an injury as diffuse if CT findings showed no mass lesion or shift of midline structures more than 5 mm, whereas we used the term *mass lesion* to describe cases of intracerebral lesion (contusion or hematoma), extracerebral lesion (subdural or epidural hematoma), or a combination of intracerebral and extracerebral lesions. The Glasgow Outcome Scale was completed at 6 mo in all disabled patients included in this study [10]. All clinical information was recorded prospectively on standard forms and entered in a computer storage file according to the data bank research protocol [9].

RESULTS

Relationship between the Duration of Coma and PTA

The duration of coma is plotted against the PTA duration for each patient in Figure 7.1. It is seen that there is a positive correlation between these intervals (Spearman rank order correlation = .44, $p < .001$), but impressive deviations from a linear relationship are also present. Eight patients who emerged from coma within 1 wk remained in PTA for more than a month after injury. In contrast, five cases with at least 20 day of coma had periods of PTA confined to less than 2 wk.

Type and Lateralization of Injury

An overall comparison of patients who sustained mass lesions (hematoma, contusion) with diffuse brain injury cases disclosed no significant difference in the duration of coma (Table 7.1). However, Table 7.1 shows a trend that approached significance for patients with a mass lesion to have a longer period of PTA than patients with diffuse injury.

To investigate the effects of lateralization of hemispheric mass lesion on the duration of coma and PTA, we searched the head injury registry of the Houston-Galveston Comprehensive Central Nervous System Injury Trauma Center for cases who had unilateral intracranial hematomas and serial GCS and GOAT scores. This search identified eight patients (seven intracerebral, one subdural) who were injured before the data bank was established. These additional cases (three left hemisphere injured, five right hemisphere injured), who were compatible with the data bank entry criteria, were included in the analysis concerning lateralization of brain injury.

Table 7.1 Age, Duration of Coma, and Posttraumatic Amnesia in Diffuse Head Injury versus Head Injury with Mass Lesions

Characteristic	Diffuse Injury		Mass Lesions		Significance of Mann-Whitney U
	Median	*Range*	*Median*	*Range*	
Number	13		37		
Age	21	10 to 51	23	10 to 59	Nonsignificant
Coma (days)	4.8	0.6 to 56.2	7.6	1.8 to 60.7	Nonsignificant
PTA (days)	5	1 to 106	13	1 to 132	$p < .06$

Note: The type of injury was inferred from CT and surgical findings. Diffuse injury implies no high density lesion and no shift of midline structures greater than 5 mm. PTA duration refers to the interval between the end of coma and first obtaining a normal orientation/memory score [4].

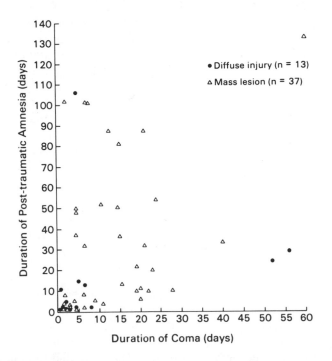

Figure 7.1 Duration of posttraumatic amnesia plotted against the duration of coma for fifty patients with severe head injuries. The presence of a high density intracranial lesion (hematoma, contusion) visualized by CT within 24 hr of injury was the criterion for a mass lesion, whereas a diffuse injury implies no evidence of such a lesion.

Preliminary analysis established that the initial GCS scores were comparable in the left hemisphere ($n=14$) and right hemisphere ($n=14$) injury groups. Analysis of the individual components of the GCS also revealed nonsignificant hemispheric differences. There was a nonsignificant trend of longer coma in the left (median = 12.6 day, range = 5 to 35) versus right (median = 7, range = 2.2 to 57.5) hemisphere mass lesion groups. The median PTA duration was 11.5 day in both the left and right hemisphere injury groups. Consistent with the overall relationship between the durations of coma and PTA (see Figure 7.1), this correlation was confirmed for patients with right hemisphere mass lesions ($r=.57$, $p<.02$) and the patients with diffuse injury ($n=13$, $r=.67$, $p<.006$). In contrast, the durations of coma and PTA were uncorrelated in patients with left hemisphere mass lesions ($r=.09$).

Duration of Impaired Consciousness in Relation to Interval before Speech

We explored the guideline proposed by Jennett and Teasdale that the duration from the time of injury to the end of PTA (in which they include both the periods of coma and severe anterograde amnesia) is approximately four times longer than the interval from injury to the restoration of speech [5]. We computed the total duration of disturbed consciousness (durations of coma and PTA) for the fifty coma data bank patients and divided this figure by the interval from the injury until the verbal score on the GCS improved to at least 3—i.e., intelligible speech. The results indicated a median ratio of 2.57; i.e., the time required for patients to achieve a normal score on a brief orientation and amnesia test was about 2.5 times longer than the delay preceding their onset of speech. The variability in this ratio was impressive, as reflected by a range from 1 to 197. The corresponding median ratios were 2.16 for the patients with diffuse injury and 2.61 for patients with mass lesions. The difference between these ratios was nonsignificant.

Duration of Impaired Consciousness in Relation to Outcome

Of the twenty-two coma data bank patients with residual disability, fifteen were rated as moderate and seven were severe according to the Glasgow Outcome Scale [10]. Consequently, these groups were combined into a single disability group for comparison with the twenty-eight coma data bank patients who achieved a good recovery. It is seen in Table 7.2 that the duration of both coma and PTA was significantly longer in the disabled group than in patients with a good recovery.

Effects of Age on Duration of Impaired Consciousness and Outcome

Comparison of the patients older than the sample median age of 23 with the younger cases disclosed a trend for a longer duration of impaired consciousness in the older group. The median duration of coma in the older patients was 9 days (range = 1 to 61) as compared to 4.8 days (range = 1 to 56) in the younger patients, a nonsignificant difference. Although older patients had a median PTA duration of 32 days (range = 1 to 132 days) as compared to 10 days in the younger group (range = 1 to 102 days), this was also nonsignificant. Table 7.2 shows that patients who achieved a good recovery were significantly younger than the patients who were still disabled at 6 mo by their injuries.

DISCUSSION

In 1932 Russell advocated adoption of the duration of disturbed consciousness (coma plus interval of severe anterograde amnesia) as a prognostic index for outcome of head injury [2]. Since the advent of a practical and reliable scale

Table 7.2 Glasgow Outcome Scale Category in Relation to Age, Duration of Coma, and Duration of PTA

Characteristic	Good Recovery		Moderate/Severe Disability		Mann-Whitney	
	Median	*Range*	*Median*	*Range*	*U*	*p*
Number	28		22			
Age	20.8	10 to 46	32.8	15 to 59	188	<.02
Coma (days)	4	0.22 to 23	10.8	1.8 to 56.7	152	<.003
PTA (days)	8	1 to 102	33.5	1.1 to 101.3	178	≤.01

to assess coma [1], neurosurgeons typically monitor the duration of coma separately from the residual period of confusion and marked amnesia. The pilot phase of the National Traumatic Coma Data Bank is the first multicenter study to monitor quantitatively the recovery of orientation and amnesia after severely injured patients emerge from coma and to study the relationship between the durations of these intervals. Although our results await confirmation in the main phase, we suggest that the relationship between coma duration and the period of PTA deviates from a linear predictive model and that a dissociation may be more common in cases with a left hemisphere mass lesion. Extrapolation from this study would predict that disproportionately long amnesia and confusion after relatively brief coma occurs in about 15% of severe nonmissile head injuries. Consistent with the impressive variability characterizing the relationship between the durations of coma and PTA in the coma data bank patients, our results provide no support for a guideline to predict the total duration of disturbed consciousness (including both coma and PTA) from the interval preceding onset of speech [5].

In view of previous reports of acute cerebral infarction [7] and intracarotid injection of sodium amytal [8] that have implicated a relationship between impaired consciousness and insult to the language-dominant hemisphere, we postulated that severely head-injured patients with unilateral left hemisphere mass lesions would exhibit a longer duration of coma than severely injured patients with right hemisphere mass lesions. Although we found a trend in the predicted direction, it was not statistically significant. Analysis of individual components of the GCS score also failed to demonstrate a significant effect for hemispheric lateralization of mass lesion. It is conceivable that concomitant diffuse or multifocal trauma to the brain in severe head injury obscures the effects of hemispheric lateralization of injury on the disturbance of impaired consciousness that has been reported for acute vascular insult [7] and intracarotid amytal injection [8].

The durations of both coma and PTA were related to the overall quality of recovery 6 mo after injury. This finding confirms previous reports [2,4,5] and indicates that the interval of PTA is prognostically useful even when it is assessed separately from coma duration. Direct measurement of PTA may be of particular prognostic importance when precise determination of coma duration is precluded because of hospital transfer or delayed evacuation. The main phase of the National Traumatic Coma Data Bank will provide an opportunity to replicate our findings.

ACKNOWLEDGMENTS

Portions of this chapter were presented at the American Association of Neurological Surgeons meeting on April 9, 1984, in San Francisco. This research was supported by Contract No. NS 3-2339, National Traumatic Coma Data Bank; Grant NS 07377, Center for the Study of Central Nervous System Injury;

and Grant NS 21889, Javits Neuroscience Investigator Award. We are grateful to Dr. Arthur L. Benton for his criticism of the manuscript and to Beverly White for manuscript preparation.

REFERENCES

1. Teasdale G, Jennett B. Assessment of coma and impaired consciousness: a practical scale. Lancet 1974;2:81–84.
2. Russell WR. Cerebral involvement in head injury. Brain 1932;55:549–603.
3. Artiola i Fortuny L, Briggs M, Newcombe F, Ratcliff G, Thomas C. Measuring the duration of post traumatic amnesia. J Neurol Neurosurg Psychiat 1980;43:377–79.
4. Levin HS, O'Donnell VM, Grossman RG. The Galveston orientation and amnesia test: a practical scale to assess cognition after head injury. J Nerv Ment Dis 1979;167:675–84.
5. Jennett B, Teasdale G. Management of head injuries. Philadelphia: F.A. Davis Company, 1981.
6. Fisher CM. Concussion amnesia. Neurology 1966;16:826–30.
7. Albert ML, Silverberg R, Reches A, Berman M. Cerebral dominance for consciousness. Arch Neurol 1976;33:453–54.
8. Serafetinides EA, Hoare RD, Driver MV. Intracarotid sodium amylobarbitone and cerebral dominance for speech and consciousness. Brain 1965;88:107–31.
9. Marshall LF, Becker DP, Bowers SA, Cayard C, Eisenberg H, Gross CR, Grossman RG, Jane JA, Kunitz SC, Rimel R, Tabaddor K, Warren J. The national traumatic coma data bank. Part 1: design, purpose, goals, and results. J Neurosurg 1983;59:276–84.
10. Jennett B, Bond M. Assessment of outcome after severe brain damage. Lancet 1975;1:480–87.

Chapter 8

Mechanisms and Management of Posttraumatic Epilepsy

L. James Willmore

One late complication of head trauma having serious medical and psychosocial impact on the patient is the development of posttraumatic epilepsy (PTE). Epilepsy is a rubric designating a condition of recurrent clinically manifest seizures that occur without cause other than an enduring physiologic abnormality of the brain. The proximate cause of PTE assumes that head trauma induces changes in the function of cortical or limbic neurons such that resultant disinhibition develops within a critical mass of cells, causing epileptiform discharges and convulsive seizures. The development of PTE initiates a cascade of events and consequences that range from the occurrence of convulsive seizures, leading to the chronic administration of anticonvulsant medication. Further, patients with epilepsy frequently experience the loss of employment, insurability, driving privileges, and self-esteem. Unlike other diseases, the treatment of epilepsy, regardless of the cause, requires a comprehensive strategy designed to control seizures, and to offer special social rehabilitation.

INCIDENCE

Population studies reveal that PTE develops within 1 yr in approximately 7% of severely injured patients hospitalized with head trauma [1]. Patients injured in combat, with a blow to the head that appears to be without neurologic significance, experience a 7% incidence of PTE, while the trauma patient with severe focal neurologic deficits develops PTE 57% of the time [2]. Missile injuries—with destruction of brain tissue and foreign body deposition within neural tissue—and hemorrhage form a subgroup with a particularly high incidence of PTE [3].

Variability in the definition of incidence is accounted for by differences in the definition of severity of injury, selection of cases based on known predictive factors, and the nature of the trauma source; combat versus civilian population. The liability to develop epilepsy appears to be related to the nature and severity of the injury or the trauma dose.

PATHOGENESIS

The pathologic changes in tissue obtained by resection of seizure foci induced by trauma include bruised parenchyma with leptomeningeal thickening, gliosis with fribrillary astrocytosis and fibrous tissue ingrowth, and neuronal rarefaction [4]. Areas of encephalomalacia, perifocal microglial reaction, and hemosiderin deposition are also observed. Head trauma with skull fracture causes diffuse gliosis of the neural parenchyma, neuronal loss, and spongiosis. Without fracture, the changes also include hemosiderin deposition. Evolution of pathologic changes from initial trauma to subsequent epileptogenesis are thought to occur [5]. It has been proposed that the early effects of trauma, including hemorrhage, edema, vascular congestion, and contusion resolve over time to form an area of gliosis, neuronal loss, and a microglial reaction [6]. Hemosiderin deposition is related to resorption of focal hemorrhage. Vascular changes include reduction in capillary number, neovascularization, and areas of ischemic necrosis with cavitation. Since the clinical and electroencephalograph (EEG) manifestations of epilepsy are not immediate in their development, it would appear that events initiated by trauma result in the development of structural or biochemical changes that may be considered as a dynamic or reactive process of epileptogenesis.

Head trauma causes direct or impact injury to the brain and may cause both delayed damage or indirect damage to neural structures [7]. Skull impact may cause skull fracture or transient skull deformation, transmission of mechanical force through the brain with a pressure wave associated with momentary cavitation and cavity collapse (cavitation bubbles), or translational or rotational effects on the brain [8]. Impact injury results in actual structural changes that include skull fracture, hematoma formation, damage to nerve fibers and blood vessels, or brain contusion or laceration. A contusion is a lesion produced by mechanical force applied to a tissue that causes the formation of an area of hemorrhage, necrosis, or actual laceration. Within the brain, shearing induced by rotational forces or transient cavitation causes bulk displacement of tissue with cellular death (necrosis) from disruption of the mechanical integrity of cells or from ischemic effects induced by macro- or microvascular injury. Hemorrhage within a contused region, typically a gyral crest, is caused by mechanical disruption of the continuity of blood vessel walls at the site of injury. Histopathologic assessment of contusions shows coagulation necrosis, edema, and hemorrhage. Late changes include cellular reactants with phagocytosis and gliosis [7].

Impact injury also causes damage to fiber tracts within the brain. Tearing of axons by mechanical forces, found most commonly in the corpus callosum, eventually results in the formation of the histopathologic changes of formation of axonal retraction balls, with reactive astrocytosis, Wallerian degeneration, and microglial star formation within a gliosed cystic lesion within white matter [7].

Delayed damage to the brain induced by the impact results in the formation of hematomas or the development of brain swelling. A hematoma developing in the subdural or epidural regions is caused by injury to large blood vessels. Intracerebral hematoma formation appears to be related to the extent and severity of coalescence of hemorrhagic contusions. Brain swelling may result from altered vasomotor regulation within regions adjacent to hemorrhages or contusions. Hypoxic injury secondary to indirect damage, status epilepticus, or ischemic cortical necrosis in arterial boundary zones from global reduction of cerebral flood flow, vasospasm, or from altered vascular autoregulation also contributes to brain swelling.

Although histopathologic changes can be identified within traumatized brain and within the trauma-induced seizure focus, the specific mechanism for posttraumatic epileptogenesis remains unknown. However, several hypotheses can be formulated, as reviewed, in part, by Jasper [6]. He proposed that extravasation of blood results in deposition of a toxic irritant within the neuropil, with induction of a reactive gliosis, ischemia, and focal alterations of the blood-brain barrier. Animal experimentation lends support to this consideration since acute [9] and chronic seizures can be induced by pial application or intracortical deposition of iron salts [10] or iron-containing blood products [11]. One potential mechanism for epileptogenesis initiated by iron-containing solutions or hemoglobin is the propagation of neural lipid peroxidation, with resultant neuronal plasma membrane changes within traumatized brain [12]. Since administration of antiperoxidants like alpha-tocopherol prevents experimental epileptogenesis induced by iron salts injection into rodent brain [12], this later hypothesis regarding lipid peroxidation warrants further evaluation.

Jasper also considered the effect of altered blood-brain barrier function on the neural ionic microenvironment [6]. Altered transport or diffusion of chemicals within blood that are normally excluded from the neural tissue within a focal brain region may change ratios of excitation/inhibition, causing seizures. He also considered the effect on seizure thresholds of altering the type and quantity of glial cells with a brain region. Of interest is the possibility that traumatic axonal damage could disrupt axonal collateral inhibition, denervate focal dendritic arborizations, or initiate aberrant resprouting with change in transmitter input to specific brain regions.

TRAUMA DOSE AND PREDICTIVE FACTORS

The severity of brain injury, reflecting trauma dose, correlates with the incidence of PTE. For example, Caveness identified six categories of head trauma based on the severity of injury [2]. Categories I to III are characterized by intact dura mater and injury causing no neurologic sequela or with obvious damage to the brain. These categories had an incidence of epilepsy from 7 to 39% respectively. If the dura was penetrated and the range of deficit was none to profound injury, then the epilepsy incidence was 20 to 57%.

The time of occurrence of the first seizure documents a latency that may be related to the injury responses of epileptogenesis. Of patients developing PTE, 63% will have had their first seizure within 1 yr, 80% by 2 yr after injury [13]. The timing of seizure may also be divided into immediate, within 24 hr; early, within the first week; or late, beyond the first week.

Although immediate seizures are defined as those occurring with the first 24 hours, 30% occur in the first hour after trauma. Patient management is complicated by immediate seizures, and posttraumatic status epilepticus by necessitating the administration of anticonvulsant medications or by causing an episode of hypoxia. An immediate seizure occasionally may be a signal event denoting the presence of an intracranial hematoma. The occurrence of an early seizure has prognostic significance for subsequent seizures. Jennett found a tenfold increase in the incidence of late epilepsy in those patients who had an early seizure [14]. Other predictive indicators associated with increased risk of late epilepsy include duration of posttraumatic amnesia beyond 24 hr, the presence of a depressed skull fracture, or the development of an intracranial hematoma. Indeed, mathematical prediction using weighted risk factors allows calculation of liability at the time of injury for development of PTE or estimation of continued risk at various times after injury [15].

The majority of patients with PTE experiences generalized convulsive seizures [16]. Secondary generalization from a focus occurs in 54% of patients, while 31% experience convulsions without any apparent prior focal activity. In Evans's series, 14% had focal seizures [13]. Complex partial seizures occur in 20% of patients in some series [16].

MANAGEMENT

Acute Seizures

A single generalized seizure occurring at the time of injury usually requires administration of a long-acting anticonvulsant, like phenytoin. Patients may be given a single loading dose of 10 to 15 mg/kg intravenously. Phenytoin must be given via a peripheral vein at a rate no greater than 50 mg/min. The patient must be monitored for bradycardia or hypotension. If these problems occur, then the rate of administration must be slowed. The drug may be diluted in 0.9% sodium chloride for purposes of loading. The daily maintenance dose of 4 to 5 mg/kg is best given as a single daily dose, either intravenously or orally. Phenytoin blood levels should be measured at the time the patient reaches steady state at 5 to 7 day after initiation of treatment. Status epilepticus can be effectively terminated by intravenous administration of 0.1 to 0.3 (up to 20 mg) mg/kg diazepam, followed by loading with phenytoin. For details on management of status, see Delgado-Esqueta et al [17].

If a patient has no further seizures other than the initial event, then critical risk factors need to be evaluated, an EEG obtained, and an assessment of ongoing risk performed. Since immediate seizures do not increase the risk of the development of PTE, consideration needs to be given to the decision to discontinue phenytoin therapy. Unfortunately, little data are available to assist the physician. A conservative approach would be to continue treatment for 1 yr after the initial seizure, obtain an EEG at that time, then taper the phenytoin dose over several months if the EEG is normal. In most states, the patient may not operate a motor vehicle for 1 yr after a genralized convulsive seizure. Driving prohibition should continue during medication withdrawal.

Early and Late Seizures

As documented, the occurrence of an early seizure is associated with an increased risk for subsequent seizure activity, identifying the patient as having PTE. Treatment initiated as described in the previous section, using 4 to 5 mg/kg of phenytoin/day, with assessment of anticonvulsant blood levels, should be continued for 5 yr after the last convulsive seizure. It could be argued that this regimen is needlessly conservative; however, no data are available to suggest that management should be otherwise. Clearly, early and complete control of seizures is associated with an increased rate of remission of PTE [18].

Late seizures should be managed by administration of an anticonvulsant selected by criteria obtained from assessment of the nature of the patient's seizure. For example, if the patient experiences generalized convulsive seizures, then phenytoin would be the drug of choice. However, if the patient has simple or complex partial seizures or generalized convulsive seizure with a focal component suggesting secondary generalization, then carbamazepine would be the drug of choice.

PHARMACOLOGIC PROPHYLAXIS

In 1972, Rapport and Penry reviewed the published reports of efforts to prevent the development of PTE by the administration of anticonvulsant medications to head-injured patients [19]. They cited three reports published by Czechoslovakian investigators. The information used in this discussion was obtained from that review.

Hoff and Hoff treated forty-eight patients with 200 mg of diphenylhydantoin; forty-six head trauma patients were not treated and served as controls. The population base used to select the study patients was not reported. At the end of this 4 yr study, 4% of the treated patients had developed epilepsy, while 38% of the controls had epilepsy. The nature of the selection of patients for entry into this study was not reported; patients were selected for inclusion into the two study groups. Anticonvulsant blood levels were not measured; hence, compliance could not be evaluated. By the time Birkmayer had reported results from this original population, and additional patients, yielding a net of 213 patients, the number of patients in each group could not be discerned from the report, but 6% of treated patients and 51% of control patients had developed epilepsy. In 1969, Popek and Musil reported similar spectacular results. They followed 87% of 167 patients for 5 yr after head injury. They treated patients with phenytoin and phenobarbital (160 to 240 mg/day and 30 to 60 mg/day respectively). At the end of this 5 yr study, none of the treated patients had epilepsy, while 21% of the controls had seizures. All these studies suffer from lack of publication of complete data to allow statistical comparisons or assessment of the total population serving at the source for the selection of patients for study. Further, anticonvulsant blood levels were not available; hence, questions of dose response and compliance could not be evaluated.

Wohns and Wyler, using a retrospective format, evaluated fifty patients treated with phenytoin and twelve patients who served as untreated controls [20]. Their base of patients for selection was 350. Of those, 120 either died or could not meet study entrance criteria. Patients lost to follow-up included 113; the number treated or not treated in that group was not reported. Blood levels of phenytoin were measured to allow maintenance of therapeutic drug levels. Ten percent of treated patients developed PTE. However, 50% of untreated control patients developed epilepsy. The study lost a very large number of patients from the selection base of 350. The study was not double blind but retrospective. The authors concluded that the hypothesis regarding prevention of the development of PTE by the administration of phenytoin was supported by their data.

An effort to improve on the deficient study designs, as noted earlier, was reported by Young et al in 1979 [21]. These authors selected eighty-four patients for a prospective study of the effect of phenytoin administration to head-injured patients selected for risk of development of PTE.

The patients received intravenous loading of phenytoin and were maintained on intramuscular or oral medication for 1 yr after injury. Striking difficulty with compliance was documented. Although the study was prospective and open, the investigators did not follow a control population of patients. At the end of 1 yr, 6% of the phenytoin-treated patients had developed seizures. The authors compared their results to the reported expected frequency of the development of PTE. A comparison of the risk factors in their patients with the percentage of patients developing PTE as derived from a literature review of patients with those same risk factors allowed them to conclude that the populations were the same. Further, given this information, they concluded that phenytoin prevented the development of PTE. This conclusion suggests that the effect of phenytoin on the process of epileptogenesis must occur very early after head injury. Further, the effect is robust since the percentage developing PTE was markedly reduced and the vast majority of the patients stopped taking phenytoin after 1 or 2 mo of compliance. An additional confounding factor noted by the authors was the uniform administration of corticosteroids to their patients whereas the historical controls did not receive those drugs.

Penry and co-workers published in abstract form the results of a 36 mo prospective, double-blind pilot study of a combination of phenobarbital and phenytoin in head trauma patients [22]. Although details were limited, they noted that the seizure probability was 21% in treated patients and 13% in the controls.

Servit and Musil reported their extensive experience with prophylactic administration of phenytoin and phenobarbital to severely injured head trauma patients [23]. The study can be assumed to be open, prospective, and at least partially controlled in nature. The minimum follow-up of their patients was 3 yr. No anticonvulsant blood levels were measured. They treated 143 patients and used 24 patients as untreated controls. The majority of patients had serial EEG studies. Over the several years of this study, 25% of the controls and 2.1% of the treated patients developed PTE.

The only prospective, double-blind, placebo-controlled study of the administration of phenytoin to head trauma patients was reported by Young et al [24]. These investigators followed 179 patients for 18 mo. They loaded patients with phenytoin and followed anticonvulsant blood levels. They followed 85 treated patients and 74 placebo control patients. At the end of the study, 12.9% of the treated patients and 10.8% of the control patients had developed PTE. Although the authors concluded that phenytoin did not prevent the development of PTE, they did suggest that a study was needed using anticonvulsant blood levels greater than 12 μg/ml before the hypothesis could be rejected.

The studies reviewed here provide conflicting conclusions. The study with the best design, equal treatment, and control populations fails to support the hypothesis that phenytoin administration will prevent the development of PTE. This rather conservative conclusion may also be evaluated within the context of the caveats, provided by Caveness et al, that warn that PTE seems to complicate the course of patients treated with phenytoin more frequently than in those patients not so treated [25]. In conclusion, the suggestion that anticonvulsant administration will somehow alter or prevent the process of epileptogenesis is not fully supported by the available data. The best approach might be to select patients in high risk categories for prophylactic administration of drugs like phenytoin.

REFERENCES

1. Annegers JF, Grabow JD, Groover RV, Laws ER, Elveback LR, Kurland LT. Seizures after head trauma: a populations study. Neurology 1980, 30:683–89.
2. Caveness WF. Epilepsy, a product of trauma in our time. Epilepsia 1976, 17:207, 215.

3. Caveness WF. Onset and cessation of fits following craniocerebral trauma. J Neurosurg 1963; 20:570–83.
4. Penfield W, Humphreys S. Epileptogenic lesions of the brain: a histologic study. Arch Neurol Psych 1940; 43:240–61.
5. Payan H, Toga M, Berard-Badier M. The pathology of posttraumatic epilepsies. Epilepsia 1970; 11:80–94.
6. Jasper HH. Physiopathological mechanisms of posttraumatic epilepsy. Epilepsia 1970; 11:73–80.
7. Lindenberg R. Tissue reactions in the gray matter of the central nervous system. In: Haymaker W, Adams RD, eds. Histology and histopathology of the nervous system. Springfield, Ill.: CC Thomas, 1982; 973–1275.
8. Lindgren SO. Experimental studies of mechanical effects in head injury. Acta Chir Scand 1966; 132 (Suppl 360):1–32.
9. Willmore LJ, Hurd RW, Sypert GW. Epileptiform activity initiated by pial iontophoresis of ferrous and ferric chloride on rat cerebral cortex. Brain Res 1978; 152:406–10.
10. Willmore LJ, Sypert GW, Munson JB. Recurrent seizures inducted by cortical iron injection: a model of posttraumatic epilepsy. Ann Neurol 1978; 4:329–36.
11. Rosen AD, Frumin NV. Focal epileptogenesis following intracortical hemoglobin injection. Exp Neurol 1979; 66:277–84.
12. Willmore LJ, Rubin JJ. Antiperoxidant pretreatment and iron-induced epileptiform discharges in the rat: EEG and histopathologic studies. Neurology 1981; 31:63–69.
13. Evans JH. Posttraumatic epilepsy. Neurology 1962; 12:665–74.
14. Jennett B. Early traumatic epilepsy. Incidence and significance after nonmissile injuries. Arch Neurol 1974; 30:394–98.
15. Feeney DM, Walker AE. The prediction of posttraumatic epilepsy. Arch Neurol 1979; 36:8–12.
16. Jennett B, Teasdale G. Neurophysical sequelae. In: Management of head injuries. Philadelphia: F.A. Davis Co., 1981;271–88.
17. Delgado-Escueta AV, Wasterlain D, Treiman DM, Porter RJ. Management of status epilepticus. NEJM 1982; 306:1337–40.
18. Walker AE. Erculei F. Posttraumatic epilepsy 15 years later. Epilepsia 1970; 11:17–26.
19. Rapport RL II, Penry JK. Pharmacologic prophylaxis of posttraumatic epilepsy: a review. Epilepsia 1972; 13:295–304.
20. Wohns RNW, Wyler AR. Prophylactic phenytoin in severe head injuries. J Neurosurg 1979;51:507–09.
21. Young B, Rapp R, Brooks WH, Madauss W, Norton JA. Posttraumatic epilepsy prophylaxis. Epilepsia 1979;20:671–81.
22. Penry JK, White BG, Brackett CE. A controlled prospective study of the pharmacologic prophylaxis of posttraumatic epilepsy. Neurology 1979;29:600–01.
23. Servit Z, Musil F. Prophylactic treatment of posttraumatic epilepsy: results of a long-term follow-up in Czechoslovakia. Epilepsia 1981;22:315–20.
24. Young B, Rapp RP, Norton JA, Haack DK, Tibbs PA, Bean JR. Failure of prophylactically administered phenytoin to prevent late posttraumatic seizures. J Neurosurg 1983;58:236–41.
25. Caveness WF, Meirowsky AM, Rish BL, Mohr JP, Kistler JP, Dillon JD, Weiss GH. The nature of posttraumatic epilepsy. J Neurosurg 1979;50:545–53.

Part II

Evoked Response Monitoring Issues

Judy R. Mackey-Hargadine
James W. Hall III

Since the 1960s, there have been dramatic advances in the measurement of sensory evoked responses (SERs). A handful of scientists in the 1960s demonstrated that cortical neural activity could be generated by sensory stimuli (sounds, electrical shocks, or flashes of light) and detected by surface electrodes at the scalp [1–6]. This electrophysiologic breakthrough was a direct result of technologic developments in instrumentation. Subsequent refinement and commercial availability of rapid, signal-averaging computers, coupled with electroencephalogram (EEG) quality physiologic measurement apparatus, led to the exciting discovery, in the early 1970s, of the so-called short-latency sensory evoked responses [7,8]. The neural activity was of very small voltage (usually several microvolts or less) and occurred within a 40 or 50 msec period following a sensory stimulus. The potentials presumably originated from subcortical and primary sensory cortical regions. Unlike the highly variable longer-latency cortical responses, the short-latency activity was typically recorded reliably, and was independent of the subject's state of arousal. Short-latency responses, e.g., were not affected by sleep, sedation, or even coma. This latter characteristic offered a distinct clinical advantage for electrophysiologic assessment of central nervous system (CNS) status in brain-injured patients.

Among the first accounts of SERs in brain injury are the experimental and clinical studies of Richard Greenberg and his colleagues in the head injury research group in Richmond, Virginia [9,10]. These investigators documented the feasibility of measuring SERs from comatose patients in an intensive care unit (ICU) environment and suggested that these electrophysiologic recordings were useful in the prediction of neurologic outcome following severe head injury [11,12]. Many others have expanded this work and introduced new applications of SER in the acute care and rehabilitation of head-injured patients [13–23]. Particularly intriguing is the possibility that evoked response

107

findings may, in some cases, be more reliable indicators of neurologic status than traditional indexes, such as clinical examination or computerized tomography (CT) [16,24].

Clinical and experimental data suggest that SERs are sensitive indicators of pathophysiologic processes affecting the CNS. A critical relationship has been established between cerebral blood flow (CBF) and alterations in the brain's electrical activity. This relationship was first documented by observing changes in the EEG during recording of CBF [25]. EEG activity was unchanged until CBF fell below 18 ml/100 gm/min. These data subsequently led to the concept of using changes in the brain's electrical activity (EEG/SER) as an indirect monitor of adequate CBF. Symon and his colleagues, using the baboon stroke model, demonstrated that alteration in the brain's CBF and somatosensory evoked response (SSER) could be linked to changes at the cellular level (e.g., potassium ion efflux and edema formation) [26,27]. Since cerebral infarction is a dynamic process—starting with synaptic failure, followed by membrane failure, and finally neuronal destruction—the reversibility of this process logically depends on early detection of subtle changes in electrical activity [27–30]. Serial monitoring appears to be the best method to detect CNS dysfunction, resulting from ischemia, before a permanent neurologic deficit occurs. Astrup reviewed the data and concluded that as long as the CBF is above 15 to 18 ml/100 gm/min, normal cellular function exists [28]. Synaptic failure occurs when the CBF drops to 10 to 15 ml/100 gm/min and membrane failure when the CBF falls to 6 to 10 ml/100 gm/min.

Data collected during intraoperative procedures suggest that EEG and evoked response parameters (latency, amplitude, morphology) may offer an electrophysiologic index of pathophysiology (such as hypoxic-ischemic events) in patients under anesthesia [31–33]. Although preliminary evidence in animal experiments suggests that development of a neurologic deficit depends on the depth of metabolic insult (e.g., ischemia, hypoxia) and on the duration of the insult, these data are not available clinically because every effort is made by the surgeon and anesthesiologist to reverse the physiologic and/or technical factors causing the insult as soon as the electrical abnormality is detected. However, clinical data do exist demonstrating that rapid changes in the SER/EEG do occur with ischemia (induced hypotension during aneurysm surgery), CNS compression (excessive retractor pressures and patient positioning), and hypoxia [30–33].

A natural extension of serial recording of SER/EEG for the early detection of CNS dysfunction is serial monitoring of brain-injured patients in the surgical intensive care unit (SICU). The first accounts of SER in brain injury were the experimental and clinical studies of Greenberg and his colleagues [9,10]. Their main theme was the feasibility of this technique in the prediction of neurologic outcome. Multimodality SER recordings in the patient's early (first 24 hr) clinical course can only predict the patient's status during that given time period. Secondary insults (hypotension, hypoxia, expanding intracranial lesions, and increasing intracranial pressure) make predicting outcome on isolated recordings during the first 2 wks extremely difficult, with one exception. The use of evoked responses in the determination of brain death, although controversial, has been established as a valuable clinical tool provided certain guidelines are followed. This concept is expanded on in Chapter 10.

Serial monitoring of SER/EEG has proven valuable in decision making in an SICU setting when neurologic evaluation and clinical assessment are impossible. The CT scan can assess the anatomical integrity of the CNS but provides no information on neurologic integrity. Recent studies have demonstrated the important application of these noninvasive bedside techniques in acute severely head-injured patients and how trends in cerebral function but no outcome can be predicted.

Multimodality SERs can be useful in defining clinical disability in the rehabilitative setting. The data indicate that there is a significant correlation between SER abnormalities and clinical disability ratings from admission to a rehabilitation unit to re-entry into the community (reviewed in Chapters 11 and 12). If a patient's disability, whether cognitive or sensory, can be identified early in the hospital course, the rehabilitation staff can develop an appropriate plan for that patient's care.

In conclusion, multimodality SER recordings appear to have exciting potential as tools for evaluation of head-injured patients from the initial acute injury period to re-entry into the community. They can provide information, through serial monitoring in the SICU, to guide the physician in decision making in complicated and neurologically unstable patients. The integrity of CNS function can be objectively measured and the success of medical or surgical management evaluated. In the rehabilitation phase, sensory and cognitive deficits have also proved to be definable, and progress can be monitored through the use of these modalities. As we learn more about CNS electrical function at the cellular level and SER recording techniques are further refined, our ability to better care for and preserve CNS function in the head injured will also improve.

REFERENCES

1. Halliday AM, Wakefield GS. Cerebral evoked potentials in patients with dissociated sensory loss. J Neurol Neurosurg Psychiat 1963;26:211–19.
2. Giblin DR. Somatosensory evoked potentials in healthy subjects and patients with lesions of the nervous system. Ann NY Acad Sci 1964;112:93–142.
3. Larson SJ, Sances A, Christenson PC. Evoked somatosensory potentials in man. Arch Neurol 1966;15:88–93.
4. Cobb WA, Dawson GD. The latency and form in man of the occipital potentials evoked by bright flashes. J Physiol (London) 1960;158:108–21.
5. Davis H, Zerlin S. Acoustic relations of the human vertex potential. J Acoust Soc Am 1966;39:109–16.
6. Walter WG. The convergence and interaction of visual, auditory and tactile response in human nonspecific cortex. Ann NY Acad Sci 1964;112:320–61.

7. Jewett DL, Romano MN, Williston JS. Human auditory evoked potentials: possible brain-stem components detected on the scalp. Science 1970;167:1517–18.
8. Jewett DL, Williston JS. Auditory-evoked far fields averaged from scalp of humans. Brain 1971;94:681–96.
9. Greenberg, RP, Becker DP. Clinical applications and results of evoked potential data in patients with severe head injury. Surgical Forum 1976;26:484–86.
10. Greenberg RP, Becker DP, Miller JD, Mayer, DJ. Evaluation of brain function in severe head trauma with multimodality evoked potentials. Part II: localization of brain dysfunction in correlation with post-traumatic neurologic condition. J Neurosurg 1977;47:163–77.
11. Greenberg RP, Newlon PG, Hyatt MS, Narayan RD, Becker DP. Prognostic implication of early multimodality evoked potentials in severely head-injured patients. A prospective study. 1981;55:227–36.
12. Newlon PG, Greenberg RP, Hyatt MS, Enas GG, Becker DP. The dynamics of neuronal dysfunction and recovery following severe head injury assessed with serial multimodality evoked potentials. J Neurosurg 1982;57:168–77.
13. Hall JW III, Huangfu M, Gennarelli TA. Auditory function in acute severe head injury. Laryngoscope 1982;92:883–90.
14. Hall JW III, Mackey-Hargadine J, Allen SJ. Monitoring neurologic status of comatose patients in the intensive care unit. In: Jacobson JJ, ed. Auditory brainstem response audiometry. San Diego: College Hill Press, 1985;254-283.
15. Seales DM, Rossiter BS, Weinstein ME. Brainstem auditory evoked responses in patients comatose as a result of blunt head trauma. J Trauma 1979;19:347–53.
16. Tsubokawa T, Nichimoto H, Yamamato T, Kitamura M, Katayama Y, Moriyasu N. Assessment of brainstem damage by the auditory brainstem response in acute severe head injury. J Neurol Neurosurg Psychiat 1980;43:1005–11.
17. Uziel A, Benezech J. Auditory brainstem response in comatose patients. Relationship with brainstem responses and level of coma. Electroencephalogr Clin Neurophysiol 1978;45:515–24.
18. Rappaport M, Hall MK, Hopkins K, Belleza T, Berrol S, Reynolds G. Evoked brain potentials and disability in brain-injured patients. Arch Phys Med Rehab 1977;58:333–38.
19. Mjoen S, Nordby HC, Torvic A. Auditory evoked brainstem responses (ABR) in coma due to severe head trauma. Acta Otolaryngol 1983;95:131–38.
20. Lutschg J, Pfenninger J, Ludin HP, Fassela F. Brain-stem auditory evoked potentials and early somatosensory evoked potentials in neurointensively treated comatose children. Am J Diseases Children 1983;137:421–26.
21. Goldie WD, Chiappa KH, Young RR, Brooks EB. Brainstem auditory and short-latency somatosensory evoked responses in brain death. Neurology 1981;31:248–56.
22. Hume AL, Cant BR, Shaw NA. Central somatosensory conduction time in comatose patients. Ann Neurol 1979;5:379–84.
23. Anziska BJ, Cracco RQ. Short latency somatosensory evoked potentials in brain dead patients. Arch Neurol 1980; 37:222–25.
24. Facco E, Martini A, Zuccarello M, Chiaranda M, Trincia G, Ori C, Giron GP. Auditory brainstem responses in post-traumatic comatose patients: assessment of brainstem damage and prognostic implications. Intensive Care Med 1983;9:194.
25. Sundt TM, Sharbrough FW, Piepgras DG, Kearns TP, Messick JM, O'Fallon WM. Correlation of cerebral blood flow and electroencephalographic changes

during carotid endarterectomy—with results of surgery and hemodynamics of cerebral ischemia. Mayo Clin Proc 1981;56:533–43.

26. Symon L, Hargadine JR, Zawirski M, Branston NM. Central conduction time as an index of ischemia in subarachnoid hemorrhage. J Neurol Sci 1979;44:95–103.

27. Astrup J, Symon L, Branston NM, Lassen NA. Cortical evoked potential and extracellular K+ and H+ at critical levels of brain ischemia. Stroke 1977;8:51–57.

28. Astrup J. Energy-requiring cell functions in the ischemic brain. Their critical supply and possible inhibition in protective therapy. J Neurosurg 1982;56:482–97.

29. Branston NM, Ladds A, Symon L, Wang AD. Comparison of the effects of ischemia on early components of the somatosensory evoked potential in brainstem, thalamus, and cerebral cortex. J Cerebral Blood Flow Metabol 1984;4:68–81.

30. Hargadine JR, Branston NM, Symon L. Central conduction time in primate brain ischemia—a study in baboons. Stroke 1980;11:637–42.

31. Raudzens PA. Intraoperative monitoring of evoked potentials. Ann NY Acad Sci 1982;388:308–26.

32. Raudzens PA, Shetter AG. Intraoperative monitoring of brain-stem auditory evoked potentials. J Neurosurg 1982;57:341–48.

33. Grundy BL. Intraoperative monitoring of sensory-evoked potentials. Anesthesiology 1983;58:72–87.

Chapter 9

Evoked Responses Monitoring in the Intensive Care Unit

Judy R. Mackey-Hargadine
James W. Hall III

Just as the operating room has expanded the application of sensory evoked response (SER) in cerebral protection, so is the intensive care unit (ICU) now proving to be another area where SER monitoring may be helpful in the evaluation of central nervous system (CNS) dysfunction. Investigators in the past have been concerned with the utilization of SERs in predicting long-term outcome based on measurements made at a single assessment soon after the injury [1,2]. In the acute phase of brain injury, a dynamic condition exists that can be influenced and modified by establishing an environment in the CNS that protects the neuron. To this end, a variety of devices have been developed to monitor physiological parameters continuously at the bedside in an attempt to prevent hypotension, hypoxia, increased intracranial pressure (ICP), and other pathophysiologic processes. However, the quality of survival of the neurons has rarely been evaluated or monitored continuously.

Experimental and clinical data exist that link changes in the SERs with acute changes in cerebral blood flow (CBF), cerebral perfusion pressure (CPP), hypoxia, ischemia, and compressive lesions [3–25]. Much of these data have been generated in the operating room during neurologic procedures. Recently, investigators have presented experimental data in the cat stroke model correlating changes in the brain's electrical activity at the cellular level with alterations in CBF and cellular metabolism [3,24,25]. These data support the concept that as the regional CBF falls to critical levels (below 16 to 18 ml/100 gm/min), the first event is synaptic failure. This failure is reflected in subtle changes in the SERs. As flow continues to fall due to either focal ischemia or systemic hypotension, membrane homeostasis fails with the initial mild efflux of potassium from the cell and edema formation followed by massive effluxes of potassium and increased edema formation. Depending on the depth and duration of ischemia, infarction of the brain may occur. At each stage in the progression toward infarction, the events can be reversed if abnormalities in the SERs (latency changes, alterations in waveform morphology, and amplitude changes) are recognized as a red flag indicating neuronal dysfunction.

Astrup recognized from his experience that when ischemia occurs, two populations of neurons exist [24]. First are those that are functionally and structurally damaged and in which recovery is limited. Second are those that are functionally damaged but structurally intact and can recover given an optimum metabolic environment. The principles that apply to the detection of neuronal dysfunction in an experimental setting and in the operating room, during neurosurgical procedures, can be applied to monitoring in the surgical ICU (SICU). Although it is a more complicated task in the SICU setting with severely head-injured patients, because of the multitude of complex interrelated parameters (ischemia, hypoxia, edema, compressive lesions, etc.), SER monitoring can be a useful technique and complementary to the other physiologic parameters monitored at bedside. In a 16 mo period, from March 1983 through July 1984, we monitored 244 patients admitted to our SICU with severe head injuries. Our experience is presented and then compared to data of other workers in the field.

Every physician involved in the care of severely head-injured patients in the SICU has faced the problem of neurologically evaluating a patient in chemical paralysis or barbiturate coma. These patients do not lend themselves to the classical neurologic evaluation, and therefore, the physician must rely on physiological parameters recorded at bedside and the CT scan. In our population, serial monitoring was carried out for a variety of reasons that were important to the medical and surgical management of these patients (Table 9.1). Since changes in the SERs can often be a subtle indicator of neuronal

Table 9.1 Clinical Factors Contributing to the Decision to Monitor CNS Status with SER's in 244 Acute, Severely Brain-injured Patients

Clinical Factor	Percent of Patients
Neurologic deterioration	66
Chemical paralysis therapy	50
High-dose barbiturate therapy	40
Determination of brain death	34
Glasgow Coma Scale score of 3 or 4 (excluding brain death)	20
Hypoxic episodes without elevated intracranial pressure (ICP)	10
Unstable ICP with a risk in transporting to CT scanner	8

Note: With some patients, the decision to monitor was based on more than one factor.

dysfunction, as discussed previously, the key to the success of SER monitoring is in early baseline studies and serial monitoring when changes in the patient's condition or parameters indicate a progressive loss of neuronal function. Intervention in the form of medical therapy, diagnostic studies, or surgical procedures can be based on the accumulated data.

METHODS

In a 16 mo period, approximately 540 patients were admitted to the Hermann Hospital SICU. Of this group 80% had an initial Glasgow Coma Scale (GCS) score of 7 or less, and 75% required ICP monitoring. SEPs were measured in 244 patients (total of 910 SEP test sessions). A majority of the patients were assessed with auditory evoked responses, [auditory brain stem (ABRs) and middle-latency (AMR) response]. Within the last 6 mos, however, somatosensory evoked responses (SSERs) were also recorded from 60 patients, usually in conjunction with the auditory modality.

With one exception, the group studied was characteristic of a severely head-injured population. Seventy percent were male. The mean age was 30 years (range of 10 to 79 years). Approximately three-fourths (76%) sustained a closed head injury in a motor vehicle accident. The remainder of the injuries were gunshot wounds, acute cerebral vascular insults, or closed head injuries secondary to falls or assault. GCS was 8 or less in 90% of the group, and 3 or 4 in 61%. The unique feature of these data, in contrast to other reports of SERs in head injury, was the average time interval between the injury and the initial SER assessment. Over 80% of the patients were transported from the scene of the injury or from an outlying hospital to the Hermann Hospital via Life Flight helicopter. This air transport system dramatically reduced transit time to the hospital and assured earlier aggressive medical management. The postinjury times of SER assessment in the group were distributed as follows: within 12 hr, 23%; within 24 hr, 48%; within 48 hr, 75%. The remainder of the patients underwent SER assessment within 2 wks, usually because of neurologic deterioration or lack of neurologic improvement.

ABR assessment was carried out with a Nicolet CA-1000/DC-2000 evoked potential system according to the following protocol. Acoustic stimuli were clicks of 0.1 msec duration presented at a rate of 21.1/sec and at an intensity level of 85 to 95 dB (normal click hearing level) with TDH-39 earphones and MX-41/AR cushions enclosed within aural domes and coupled to circumaural cushions. Stimuli were presented monaurally to the right and left ears. The ABR was detected with gold cup electrodes. The positive voltage electrode was at a high forehead, midline location, the negative voltage (earclip) electrode was on the stimulated ear, and the ground electrode was at a low forehead location. In addition to this standard electrode array, simultaneous four-channel ABR recordings were made with all patients in an attempt to clarify wave form morphology [18]. The neural signal was amplified (x 100,000) and filtered at

30 to 3,000 Hz, whenever possible, or 150 to 3,000 Hz if low frequency artifact was present. A minimum of 512 sample points was used. Interelectrode impedance was always less than 5,000 ohm. ABR data were analyzed and interpreted by the second author (JWH) without knowledge of CBF outcome.

SSERs were stimulated and averaged with a Neurotrac (Interspec) instrument. Stimuli were 1,000 electrical pulses of 0.1 msec duration delivered to the median nerve of each arm at a rate of 4.1/sec. Neural activity was detected with a dual channel, subcutaneous needle electrode (Grass) recording array. One channel employed a negative voltage electrode over the stimulus ipsilateral ERB's point (supraclavicular) and a positive voltage forehead electrode. With the second channel, the negative voltage electrode was located over the parietal cortex contralateral to the stimulated side, and the positive voltage electrode was on the forehead. A large, disk-type ground electrode was placed on the proximal forearm on the stimulated side. Neural activity was amplified (x 100,000) and band-pass filtered (5 to 1,500 Hz) before the averaging process. Interelectrode impedance was always less than 5,000 ohm. SSER data were interpreted by the first author (JMH).

CASE REPORTS

Case 1: SERs and Surgical Therapy

A 32-year-old male fell approximately 8 ft from a scaffolding, struck his occiput, and was immediately unconscious. He was taken to a local emergency room, where he was reported to be following commands. Following a grand mal seizure, the patient became unresponsive, with a right fixed and dilated pupil. He was intubated and transported to Hermann Hospital via Life Flight. En route his GCS was 4. On arrival at the emergency center 2 hrs post injury, neurologic examination showed the right pupil dilated and unreactive and the left pupil sluggishly reactive. Corneal reflex was present. Painful stimulus produced a decerebrate motor response on the right and a purposeful response on the left.

An emergency CT revealed a large epidural hematoma in the right temporal area extending to the parietal region with a moderately severe midline shift from right to left. There was a hemorrhagic contusion in the left frontal region. The perimesencephalic cistern was obliterated, suggesting transtentorial herniation. The patient was immediately taken to the operating room where he underwent a craniotomy to remove the epidural hematoma and to place an ICP monitor. The patient was transferred to the SICU. Opening ICP in the SICU was 40 mm Hg. GCS was 6. ABR assessment at that time (9 hrs post injury) showed a well-formed and reliably recorded ABR and AMR bilaterally (Figure 9.1). Medications included mannitol, dexamethasone, diphenylhydantoin, and a paralyzing agent (metacurine). With the patient in coma and

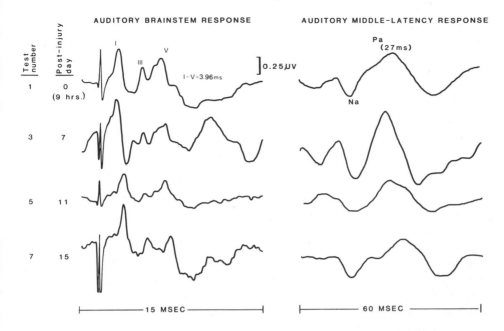

Figure 9.1   Serial ABR and AMR recordings (right ear stimulation) for a 32-yr-old male with severe closed head injury (Case 1). Findings were bilaterally symmetrical.

chemically paralyzed, normal ABRs and AMRs provided an additional parameter to aid us in following the patient's neurologic progress.

The patient's hospital course during the following 17 days was complex for both the patient and neurosurgeon. Initially, he improved neurologically. Three days post injury, GCS had improved from 6 to 10, and he was moving all extremities without a deficit. His ABRs and AMRs remained normal bilaterally. However, a CT scan that day (routine follow-up) revealed a large extracerebral hematoma in the right temporoparietal region associated with the area of the previous epidural hematoma. Another new CT finding was a small hemorrhagic contusion involving the brain stem, along the tentorial edge on the right. The ICP was controlled with mannitol, chemical paralysis, and hyperventilation. By the sixth postinjury day, he was following commands, although he remained lethargic, with no neurologic deficits except an incomplete third nerve palsy and a sixth nerve palsy. His ICP was under control with minimum medications, his ABRs and AMRs remained normal, and his neurologic status had stabilized with no major deficits except residual third and sixth nerve palsies. Surgery to remove the reaccumulated right epidural hematoma was delayed until his pulmonary status had improved. However, the following day he developed documented sepsis with a temperature of 41°C and intermittent hypotension (mean arterial pressure to 70 mm Hg). Neurologic status was unchanged (evaluated when chemical paralysis was reversed), and ICP was controlled with mannitol, metacurine, and morphine. The ABR remained normal although AMR amplitude was reduced, perhaps due to the effect of morphine. An attempt to rescan the patient was abandoned because his ICP increased to 45 mm Hg when his head was lowered, and it was not immediately responsive to a mannitol bolus.

In the next 2 to 3 days, there was some evidence of resolution of this reduced cerebral compliance. Unfortunately, his pulmonary problems and sepsis worsened. He began resisting ventilation, and ICP spikes to 50 mm Hg were recorded. Increased muscle paralysis and sedation were required, and valid neurologic assessment was therefore not possible. Throughout this period, serial SER measurements yielded a normal ABR and AMR bilaterally (see Figure 9.1). With reversal of paralysis/sedation, the patient was alert and responsive to relatives with no focal deficits except the residual right third nerve and left sixth nerve palsy. As illustrated in Figure 9.1, a normal ABR and AMR were again consistently recorded during these rather difficult 2 wks post injury. Subtle alterations in AERs were observed only in the eleventh postinjury day. These were associated with a transient reduction in mean arterial pressure to 76 mm Hg (CPP of 60 mm Hg).

Seventeen days post injury, ICP was stable without medication. The patient was following (eye[E], motor [M], vocal [V]) commands [GCS 9/$E_3M_6V_1$ (still intubated)], but he had developed a mild left hemiparesis. The next day he was taken to the operating room for the removal of an epidural hematoma and placement of a right frontal bone window for ultrasound measurements and a left frontal subarachnoid ICP monitor. Over the next few days his ICP remained normal and his hemiparesis cleared. His only problem remained intermittent pulmonary infections. He was transferred out of SICU with a GCS of 15. When placed in a rehabilitation facility 50 days after injury, the patient was communicating and prognosis for return to employment was good.

Comment

Initially, CT findings were grossly abnormal and suggested transtentorial herniation. There were marked neurologic deficits. Prognosis appeared poor. The patient recovered his first surgical intervention, but his postoperative course was plagued by recurrence of the epidural hematoma, pulmonary and ICP complications, and sepsis. Consistently normal AER findings contributed to the decision to postpone surgery and repeat CT scanning until these problems were resolved. The ABR showed no evidence of rostral brain stem dysfunction, and the AMR was likewise repeatedly normal, providing electrophysiologic evidence of cortical functional integrity in the temporal lobe region, despite CT evidence of gross cerebral pathology and unstable ICP. Although the presence of a normal ABR does not imply good prognosis, the consistently normal AMR was considered an indication of good neurologic and communicative outcome [16,17]. In this stage, medical and surgical decisions were not based on the AERs alone; however, there were periods in the patient's hospitalization when they were the only parameter available to follow cerebral function.

Case 2: SERs and Medical Therapy

The patient was a 17-year-old male who sustained a severe head injury when he fell out of the trunk of a moving automobile. At the scene, he was responsive, with purposeful movement to pain. Within 45 mins after the accident, the patient was transported via Life Flight helicopter to Hermann Hospital Emergency Center. He was extremely agitated on arrival, and a neurologic examination could not be carried out. Within 30 mins, however, pupils were found to be 3 mm, midposition, and sluggishly reactive to light bilaterally. GCS was 7. Emergency CT showed a left frontal hemorrhagic contusion and a subarachnoid hemorrhage. Ventricles were within normal limits. A midline brain stem (upper pons and midbrain) hemorrhage was noted. The patient was taken to the operating room for placement of an ICP monitor and then was taken to SICU. In the first 2 hrs post injury, ICP became elevated (to 33 mm Hg), requiring aggressive hyperventilation, sedation, and paralysis. ICP responded well to a bolus of mannitol. Neurologic status remained unchanged. Positive corneal and oculocephalic (doll's eyes) reflexes were observed.

Brain stem and cortical AERs, initially assessed within 12 hrs post injury, were normal bilaterally. ABR data are related to physiologic parameters and hospital course in Figure 9.2. Over the course of the first 5 days post injury, elevated ICP (to 40 mm Hg) was a persistent problem despite aggressive management with the noted therapy. Since the patient met our criteria for barbiturate coma, barbiturates were started. On postinjury day 6, barbiturate blood level was 25 mg/ml. Ultrasound on that day revealed a subtle left-to-right shift. There was an abnormal prolongation of rostral brain stem transmission by ABR. The right pupil was still 3 mm and sluggishly reactive, but the left pupil was 3 mm and now briskly reactive. By the ninth postinjury day, ICP was consistently in the low 20s and increased directly with increases in mean arterial pressure (MAP). The following morning (10 A.M.), rostral ABR responses continued to be abnormal, with normal caudal brain stem transmission time bilaterally. Later in the day (2 P.M.), the patient's pupils became fixed and dilated. Continuous ABR monitoring during this period revealed a worsening of the rostral ABR latency abnormality and the development of delayed caudal brain stem transmission time. Throughout this ABR testing the ICP did not exceed 13 mm Hg; however, the CPP ranged from 64 to 68 mm Hg (versus greater than 80 mm Hg on most previous assessments). Improvement of CPP through elevation of the systemic MAP significantly improved the abnormalities in the ABR responses. A normal appearing AMR was consistently recorded bilaterally.

Two weeks postinjury, neurologic status was improved. Pupils were 2 mm

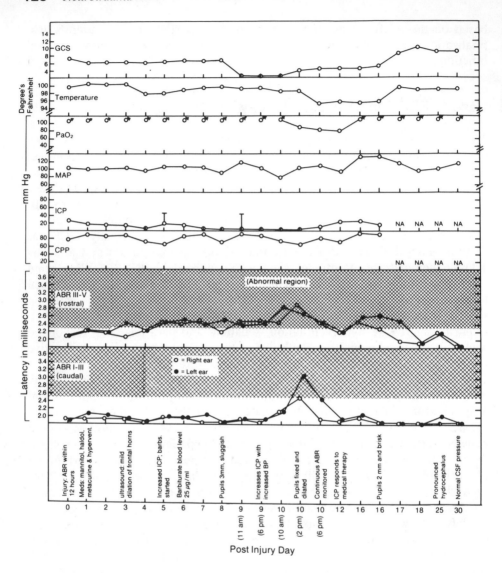

Figure 9.2   Chronologic summary of physiologic and ABR data for a 17-yr-old male with severe closed head injury (Case 2).

and briskly reactive bilaterally. The GCS was artificially low due to the intermittent need for chemical paralysis and sedation. ICP continued to be dependent on the blood pressure and usually was in the 20s. ABR abnormalities had reversed, and all responses (ABR and AMR) were within normal limits bilaterally. On the sixteenth postinjury day, rostral ABR abnormalities were again recorded. Medication for hypertension was begun, with a resulting decrease in

ICP (to less than 20 mm Hg) and a second reversal of ABR rostral abnormalities (Figure 9.3). However, as the MAP dropped from 100 mm Hg to 82 mm Hg (1:20 P.M.), the ABR wave I to V latency (brain stem transmission time) was significantly prolonged by 1.20 msec. The ICP remained within normal range. With a reliably recorded ICP in the normal range and a CPP of 79 mm Hg, evidence of dysfunction (abnormal wave components I to V latency) led us to question loss of autoregulation and to consider ischemia as the basis of dysfunction. Because of the previous changes in ABR associated with decreases in MAP, a decision was made to elevate the MAP and continuously monitor the brain stem with ABR. Elevation of the MAP resulted in improvement of

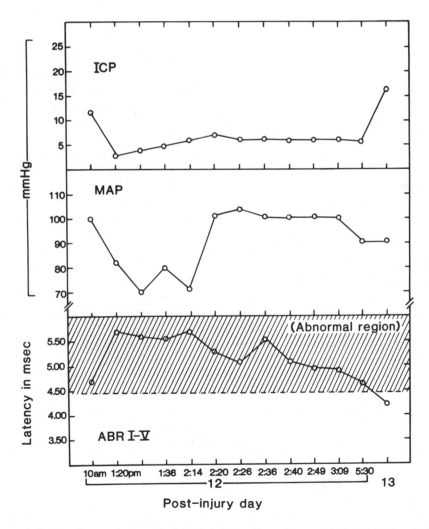

Figure 9.3   Continuously recorded ABR data for Case 2 correlated with ICP and MAP.

the ABR (2:20 P.M.) with virtually no change in the ICP. Stabilization of the MAP at 100 mm Hg produced a progressive improvement in the wave I to V latency, approaching normal values by 5:30 P.M. The ICP during the period of MAP manipulation remained unchanged, as did the patient's other physiologic parameters. These data indicated that the brain stem was subject to ischemic changes when the MAP decreased below 100 mm Hg and that brain stem dysfunction can exist in the presence of a normal ICP. With particular attention being directed to maintaining a MAP in the 90 to 100 mm Hg range over the next few days, the patient's neurologic status improved: after 3 mos of hospitalization, he was transferred to a rehabilitation facility. He was discharged from the rehabilitation hospital 2 mos after admission to be followed as an outpatient.

Comment

Patients admitted with CT evidence of cerebral and brain stem pathology are often at risk for further ischemic events. The therapy (chemical paralysis and/ or barbiturate coma) needed to protect brain function can abolish critical neurologic parameters that are important predictors of impending CNS dysfunction. This is especially true when the physician is recording a normal ICP and acceptable physiologic parameters. Loss of autoregulation in this patient could have been predicted from his early hospital course because the ICP followed the trend of the MAP. It is well documented that following ischemic episodes, a period of time exists when select areas of the brain are at considerable risk following small drops in MAP [3,4,5,23,24,25]. Neurons that are not structurally damaged but functionally injured (synaptic or membrane failure) are at greatest risk due to regional loss of autoregulation.

In this patient, significant abnormalities in the ABR were reversed with aggressive medical treatment on two separate occasions; one associated with hypertension and the other associated with hypotension. At one point the pupils became fixed and dilated with no deterioration of the ABR or AMR. Based on evoked potential evidence of CNS integrity, aggressive medical therapy and serial ABR monitoring were continued.

Early herniation does not inevitably lead to brain stem dysfunction and can be reversed with a favorable outcome. The ABR allows a method of evaluating the degree of dysfunction and the degree of success or lack of success with various medical treatments. Particular attention to the ABRs interwave latencies may help in diagnosis of the precipitating factor. Abnormality in the III to V interwave latency (rostral brain stem) appears to be indicative of early uncal herniation or midbrain structural lesions, even in the absence of pupillary changes. A process that affects the entire auditory brain stem transmission time (increase in the I to V interwave latency) could be the result of a metabolic (hypoxia), structural (acute hydrocephalus or the end stage of herniation), or ischemic event. On day 12 post injury in this patient, a significant increase in the I to V interwave latency was associated with a normal ICP and a decrease in the MAP (CPP of 68 mm Hg). Serial ABR monitoring during elevation of the MAP demonstrated a reversal of the I to

V wave abnormality and the conclusion that the brain stem was subject to ischemia at lower MAP, probably on the basis of loss of autoregulation. Although AER monitoring can not define a definite cause of brain stem dysfunction, it can be a useful parameter in the identification of pathophysiologic events requiring management and in evaluating the success of medical and/or surgical therapy, especially when ICP is normal.

Case 3: Identification of Vascular Lesions

A 32-year-old male was involved in a motor vehicle accident and sustained a severe anterior chest injury. In the emergency room, the patient was neurologically intact with a GCS of 15. He was hypoxic (PO_2 = 60 mm Hg) and hypotensive (systolic blood pressure of 66 mm Hg). In the SICU, his postintubation PO_2 was 65 mm Hg and PCO_2 was 56. On day 1 post injury, he was taken to the operating room for a thoracotomy. His GCS remained 15. The following day, adequate oxygenation continued to be a problem, with the PO_2s ranging from 62 to 91 mm Hg. That evening the patient's neurologic status worsened and he became unresponsive. Pupils were 6 mm bilaterally and nonreactive to light. A CT scan demonstrated a right hemispheric infarct with a 2 cm right-to-left shift. An ICP monitor was placed, with an opening pressure of 40 mm Hg. He was aggressively managed medically to control his ICP.

The following day, ABRs (Figure 9.4) were obtained with the anticipation of declaring the patient brain dead, since clinically he met criteria of brain death. The ABRs recorded following right ear stimulation were normal. With left ear stimulation, an abnormality was noted in the III to V interwave latency (rostral brain stem). The ABRs appeared remarkably good compared to the CT scan. In reviewing the history of the patient, there was no indication that the patient had sustained a head injury; his only injury was a steering wheel injury to the anterior chest wall. The question was raised as to whether a carotid artery injury with delayed occlusion could have accounted for the hemispheric infarct. A nuclear cerebral perfusion scan demonstrated no flow through the right carotid artery but good flow through the left carotid artery. The hypoxia and hypotension early in the patient's hospital course probably contributed to the ischemia and resulting edema leading to infarction. Despite aggressive control of the ICP, the patient did poorly and ABRs recorded approximately 24 hr later demonstrated no brain stem function (refer to Figure 9.4), and a follow-up nuclear cerebral perfusion study demonstrated no cerebral flow.

Comment

This case was instructive for several reasons. It pointed out the need for early identification of vascular lesions in the carotid and basilar systems in patients at risk. Even though a patient is awake with a GCS of 15, as this patient was,

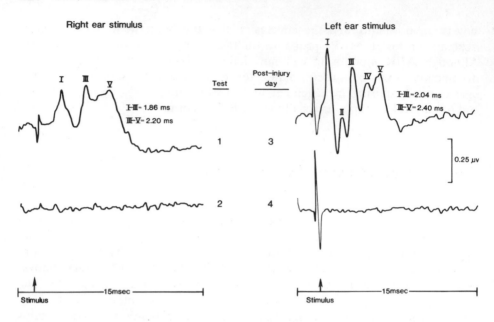

Figure 9.4   Serial ABR recordings for a 32-yr-old male with a severe anterior chest injury sustained in a motor vehicle accident (Case 3).

there is still the possibility of a vascular injury that could be potentially lethal if not promptly detected. SERs can be extremely helpful in this setting. SSERs are now being used to detect early ischemia in patients with carotid artery occlusive lesions and intracerebral aneurysms yet no neurologic deficits. Since cerebral angiography cannot be done with all patients who are neurologically intact but by the nature of their injury are at risk for a carotid artery injury, SSERs may provide a simple noninvasive technique for screening these patients.

Recently, we confirmed in a 19-year-old motor vehicle accident patient a small basilar artery thrombosis on angiography that was associated with an abnormal ABR. Normal ABRs were recorded on admission, but over a 3 day period a unilateral delay in brain stem transmission developed. The patient was improving, but unilateral deterioration in her ABRs raised the question of early brain stem ischemia. An angiogram was ordered to evaluate the posterior circulation, and the thrombosis in the basilar artery was identified. She was placed on heparin and over the next few days the ABR returned to normal. Although the clinical exam did not indicate brain stem ischemia, the progressive unilateral prolongation of the ABR was taken as evidence that a brain stem lesion did exist. With a normal CT of the posterior fossa, a vascular lesion had to be ruled out. Vascular occlusions of the carotid and basilar arteries may result from trauma. However, most of these lesions have been identified only after a neurologic event has occurred. With the identification of risk factors (facial fractures, chest injuries, hyperextension injuries, etc.) and screening with SER monitoring, vascular occlusions may be detected earlier in patients with neurologic deficits, with a subsequent decrease in the associated morbidity.

Case 4: SERs in Barbiturate Coma

A 12-year-old girl was involved in an automobile-train accident. She was admitted to the Hermann Hospital emergency room with a severe closed head injury. GCS was 6. Emergency CT scan showed diffuse brain edema without a midline shift and air in the basal cistern. The ICP opening pressure was normal. Twelve hours later, however, in the SICU, ICP became elevated and required mannitol, morphine, metacurine, and high dose barbiturates to control it. A total of nine AER assessments were carried out, beginning on the third postinjury day. A normal ABR was consistently recorded, but there was no AMR presumably due to the barbiturates. To monitor neurologic status further in barbiturate coma, serial SSERs and compressed spectral array (CSA) EEG activity were measured (Figure 9.5). From postinjury days 3 through 6, barbiturate blood levels were in the 32 to 67 μg/ml range. The patient was well oxygenated and normothermic. Pupils were 6 to 7 mm and not reactive to light. Brain stem signs were not apparent. During barbiturate coma the EEG was isoelectric (see the right portion of Figure 9.5). On day 3, there was a small amplitude, but reliably recorded, SSER (left side, Figure 9.5). Central conduction times (CCT) were significantly prolonged bilaterally (9.77 msec left, 9.38 msec right); however, the interhemispheric difference (IHD) remained normal (less than 0.6 msec). Although the ICP was normal (16 mm Hg), CPP was low (48 mm Hg). Since barbiturates are reported to have no serious effect on the short-latency SSERs [26,27], the bilateral prolongation of the SSERs was presumed to be the result of cerebral ischemia due to the low CPP. Repeat SSER testing in the next 3 days revealed a progressive increase in CCTs bilaterally (e.g., from 9.4 msec to 12.1 msec for the right cortex) that appeared to be associated with persistently low CPPs. The ICP throughout this period remained within a normal range (6 to 17 mm Hg). Waveform morphology of the SSER showed some deterioration, but the N20 peak latency was easily identified and readily reproducible. This disorganization of waveform morphology presumably reflects the effects of ischemia on synaptic function [24]. By 1 wk post injury, the patient was no longer in barbiturate coma. There was electrophysiologic evidence of improving CNS function, including CSA-EEG activity; a bilateral decrease in CCT (to 9 msec) and increased amplitude and organization of the SSER waveform morphology; and a well-formed AMR. During the remainder of the patient's hospital course, she continued to improve and was discharged home after a period of rehabilitation.

Comment

Barbiturate coma demolishes the neurologic examination, but the short-latency SEPs offer a clinically feasible means of monitoring neurologic status and

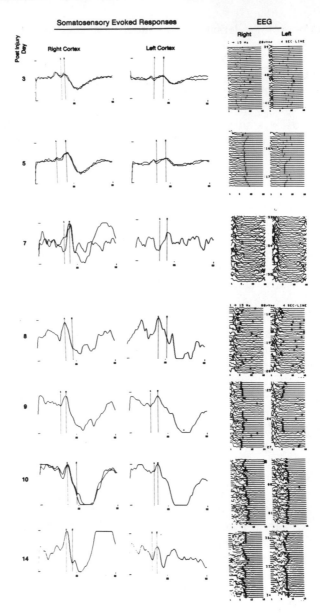

Figure 9.5   Serial SSER and compressed spectral array electroencephalography (CSA-EEG) recordings for a 12-yr-old female with a severe closed head injury (Case 4).

assessing the effectiveness of medical management. The ABR is resistant to the effect of barbiturates. The SSER is apparently influenced only by extremely high blood levels (at least based on animal studies), and there is little, if any, effect on SSER at levels needed to induce barbiturate coma clinically. In combination, these SERs, therefore, can contribute to documentation of brain stem and cerebral functional status in barbiturate coma. Deterioration or improvement of SER findings can be attributed to neurologic changes.

In Case 4, changes were noted in the SSER as the CPP decreased even though the ICP remained normal, and these changes were reversed with elevation of the CPP at the termination of barbiturate coma. With case 3 changes in SSER waveform morphology occurred in the setting of barbiturate coma with a decrease in ICP (34 to 20 mm Hg). Aggressive treatment with mannitol resulted in an improvement of SSER waveform morphology, a decrease in ICP, and an increase in CPP. Treatment of cerebral dysfunction resulting from severe head injury is a complex problem because we have not fully answered the question of how ICP and CPP interrelate to cause CNS dysfunction. The CSA-EEG provides an electrophysiologic index of the adequacy of barbiturate dosage; that is, a therapeutic dose is expected to suppress the EEG (as shown in Figure 9.5). The SERs, in contrast, can provide electrophysiologic data when the EEG is suppressed and the CNS is at maximum risk because of an unstable and uncontrollable ICP. The need for this application of SERs and CSA-EEG is not uncommon, as barbiturate therapy is not uncommonly used with acute severely head-injured patients.

DISCUSSION

The complex problem of the medical and surgical management of the severely head-injured patient has had a critical impact on hospital and medical resources. With advances in critical care technology and transportation resource systems (helicopter versus ground transportation from the accident scene), patients who would have died at the scene or during ground transportation are surviving until they reach the emergency room. Physicians involved in the decision to resuscitate the severely head-injured patient are faced with a new ethical problem. Legal guidelines have been proposed in many states for declaring the patient brain dead (see Chapter 10). However, once the decision for full resuscitation has been made, the goal of surgical and medical management has to be the protection of CNS function. CT has allowed us to identify anatomical lesions, but just how these lesions affect cerebral electrical function has not been fully explored. With the advent of SER/EEG monitoring in the SICU, we are making progress toward that end.

The original clinical experience with multimodality SER measurements by Greenberg and his colleagues centered around the analysis of the longer-latency SERs in the prediction of outcome [1,2]. With experience, other investigators have expanded this concept and, more important, realized that the short-latency ABR and SSER were better suited for analysis because of their resistance to many of the commonly used agents (morphine and barbiturates) in the treatment of brain-injured patients, as well as the deep level of coma observed.

Whether SERs acquired in the acute phase of cerebral dysfunction are analyzed with a structured grading system or according to latency, amplitude, or waveform morphology, as we have reported, attention must also be given to the other physiological parameters if SERs are to play an important part in management. As with any new technical advance, care has to be exerted in interpretation of SERs in isolation until more experience has been gained in the clinical setting. There is experimental evidence that the ABR and SSEP change with ischemia and increased ICP, with and without evidence of trans-tentorial herniation [14–17,21,22]. Clinically, the data are much more difficult to interpret because of varying methodology and inpatient variability. However, certain conclusions recur in most studies. First, normal brain stem ABR components in the acute phase are not correlated with survival [16,17]. When the long-, middle-, and short-latency components are preserved, patients have a substantially better chance of survival [1,2,16,28,29]. In barbiturate coma, if the AMR is recorded prior to coma and reappears following withdrawal of barbiturate coma, outcome appears improved [1,2]. One must be leery of the problems of eighth nerve damage due to basilar fractures and middle ear effusions as a source of an absent ABR in the face of intact brain stem signs [30]. As we point out in Chapter 10, "the apparent high proportion of patients yielding no response . . . cannot be confidently used as evidence of brain stem dysfunction since it may reflect, instead, serious peripheral otologic pathology." This problem can be partially overcome by early serial ABR testing.

Progressive deterioration of the ABR, especially in a rostral-caudal fash-ion, may be correlated with unilateral or bilateral pupillary dilation [1,2,31,32]. With early detection of an abnormal III to V ABR interwave latency, reversal of the abnormality is possible prior to the development of pupillary changes (see Case 3). An abnormal ABR in conjunction with normal ICP has been described by Anderson et al, with the patients having an unfavorable outcome more often than a favorable one [28]. These investigators attributed the lack of the expected relationship between ICP and neurologic outcome to a com-bination of factors including the method of ICP monitoring (bolt versus ven-triculostomy), age of the patient, and primary intracranial process (intracranial mass lesion). However, they did not seem to consider brain stem ischemia as a contributing factor. With loss of autoregulation, episodes of relatively mild hypotension can further damage a brain stem already at risk (see Case 2). We were perplexed by the presence of abnormal ABRs in patients with normal ICP and no CT evidence of structural brain stem lesions until serial SER monitoring during blood pressure manipulation (other physiological parameters held constant) demonstrated reversal of the ABR prolongation. It appears that serial monitoring of ABRs may play an important role in the detection and protection of the brain stem from ischemic events, when all other parameters appear normal. Finally, the results of Rosenberg's study [29], as well as early work by Starr and his group [33], indicate that the ABR must be interpreted in light of the cause of coma. In their experiences, in contrast to the patients in coma due to severe head trauma, survival after coma due to anoxic insults could not be related to the presence of normal brain stem components. Therefore, interpretation of the ABRs and AMRs is not always straightforward and is often complex, but the findings can be useful in management and predicting outcome.

The SSER central pathway (median nerve stimulation) provides further access in exploring dysfunction in the CNS. While the middle-and long-latency SSERs are sensitive to the same factors that affect the longer-latency AERs, the short-latency SSERs are relatively resistant to deep levels of coma, and according to Hume and Cant [26], phenobarbital contributes only a 4% variance in the CCT. However, in SSER testing carried out on patients in barbiturate coma, abnormal CCTs should be interpreted cautiously, and analysis should include not only latency but also waveform morphology and amplitude. Data indicate that the SSER is much more resistant to high barbiturate levels than EEG [27]. Therefore, it is possible during barbiturate coma to follow cortical activity with SSERs even when the EEG is isoelectric.

SSERs have been analyzed as the sole evoked potential measurement and in combination with ABRs to evaluate neuronal dysfunction in patients with head injuries and coma due to metabolic causes [1,2,16,17,28,29,31,33, 34,35]. It is difficult to compare results of these various studies. Differences among the studies include the systems used for evoked potential grading, the interval from the time of head injury or onset of coma and initial evoked potential testing, and the etiology of brain injury for the patient populations studied. However, encouraging conclusions are common to most studies. Normal SSERs recorded from the cortex in the acute and subacute phase of coma are usually correlated with a favorable outcome. Loss of a cortical response, either unilaterally or bilaterally, was associated with a less favorable outcome [1,2,26,28]. Consideration must be given in the interpretation of an absent or distorted SSER to the influence of brain stem and thalamic lesions in the presence of retained cortical function. Confirmation of brain stem lesions on CT are not always possible except with the newer generation of CT scanners. Analysis of ABR measurements, in combination with SSER analysis, will probably assist in our understanding and interpretation of SSER abnormalities.

Despite the various approaches to the utilization of SERs in evaluation of the severely head-injured patient, they present some exciting new directions for clinical application. First, they show promise as a monitor of medical and surgical management in the SICU. Second, they may help in the understanding of the pathophysiologic mechanisms of brain injury. Presumably, these pathophysiologic events (hypoxia, ischemia, edema, increased ICP) differentially influence the various SER neuroanatomic and neurophysiologic substrates because of differences in metabolic requirements, neuron populations, and blood supply. The duration and number of insults that various areas of the CNS can tolerate and still recover from are unknown. Investigation of these complex interactions among pathophysiology and the SERs would have readily apparent clinical application and long-term implications for the management of severe brain injury. Third, there is an important and well-recognized need for increased knowledge correlating CT evidence of structural damage with evidence of neuronal dysfunction.

Our clinical experience with serial SER measurements in over 244 comatose brain-injured patients can be summarized as follows:

1. Valid SER recordings within hours of injury are feasible at bedside in the SICU and are especially valuable if SER testing is to be meaningfully incorporated with other physiological parameters in patient management.
2. Short-latency SERs appear to be independent of depth of coma, including deep barbiturate-induced coma.
3. Changes in SER latency and waveform morphology can be correlated with dynamic pathophysiology in head injury, such as hypoxia, increased ICP, and increased CPP.
4. SER abnormalities, especially the ABR, may precede other clinical evidence of neurologic deterioration and can occur in the presence of normal ICP.
5. Reversible SEP abnormalities in brain injury have been associated with effective surgical and/or medical management.
6. As suggested by Starr [33] and discussed by Hall and Hargadine in Chapter 10, the SER can be effectively applied in the determination of brain death and offers an objective and cost-effective measure of brain stem and cortical integrity that is not influenced by intoxicants and CNS depressants, unlike the clinical examination.

As our technology develops and clinical experience increases, the use of SERs in protection of CNS function may advance to the status of, e.g., electrocardiogram monitoring of cardiac status.

REFERENCES

1. Greenberg RP, Becker DP, Miller JD, Mayer, DJ. Evaluation of brain function in severe head trauma with multimodality evoked potentials. Part II: localization of brain dysfunction in correlation with posttraumatic neurologic condition. J Neurosurg 1977;47:163–77.
2. Greenberg RP, Newlon PG, Hyatt MS, Narayan RD, Becker, DP. Prognostic implication of early multimodality evoked potentials in severely head-injured patients. A prospective study. J Neurosurg 1981;55:227–36.
3. Branston NM, Ladds A, Symon L, Wang AD. Comparison of the effects of ischaemia on early components of the somatosensory evoked potentials in brainstem, thalamus, and cerebral cortex. J Cereb Blood Flow Metab 1984;4:68–81.
4. Hargadine JR, Branston NM, Symon L. Central conduction time in primate brain ischaemia—a study in baboon. Stroke 1980;11:637–42.
5. Hargadine JR. Intraoperative monitoring of sensory evoked potentials. In: Rand R, ed. Microneurosurgery. St. Louis: Mosby 1985;92-112.
6. Jones TH, Morawetz RB, Crowell RM, Marcoux RW, FitzGibbon SJ, DeGirolami

U, Ojemann RG. Thresholds of focal cerebral ischemia in awake monkeys. J Neurosurg 1981;54:773–82.

7. Eisenberg HM, Turner JW, Teasdale G, Rowan J, Feinstein R, Grossman RG. Monitoring of cortical excitability during induced hypotension in aneurysm operations. J Neurosurg 1979;50:595–602.

8. Raudzens PA. Intraoperative monitoring of evoked potentials. Ann NY Acad Sci 1982;388:308–26.

9. Grundy BL. Intraoperative monitoring of sensory-evoked potentials. Anesthesiology 1983;58:72–87.

10. Sutton LN, Bruce DA, Welsh F. The effects of cold-induced brain edema and white-matter ischemia on the somatosensory evoked response. J Neurosurg 1980;53:180–84.

11. Lesnick JE, Michele JJ, Simeone FA, DeFeo S, Welsh FA. Alteration of somatosensory-evoked potentials in response to global ischemia. J Neurosurg 1984;60:490–94.

12. Carter LP, Yamagata S, Erspamer R. Time limits of reversible cortical ischemia. Neurosurgery 1983;12:620–23.

13. Little JR, Lesser RP, Lueders H, Furlan AJ. Brain stem auditory evoked potentials in posterior circulation surgery. Neurosurgery 1983;12:496–502.

14. Kraus N, Ozdamar O, Heydemann PT, Stein L, Reed NL. Auditory brain-stem responses in hydrocephalic patients. J Electroencephalogr Clin Neurophysiol 1984;59:310–17.

15. McPherson D, Blanks J, Foltz E. Intracranial pressure effects on auditory evoked response in the rabbit: preliminary report. Neurosurgery 1984;14:161–66.

16. Hall JW III, Mackey-Hargadine JR. Auditory evoked responses in severe head injury. Seminars in Hearing 1984;5:313–36.

17. Hall JW III, Mackey-Hargadine JR, Allen SJ. Monitoring neurologic status of comatose patients in the intensive care unit. In: Jacobson JJ, ed. Auditory brainstem response audiometry. San Diego: College Hill Press, 1985;254–83.

18. Bennett MH, Maurice JA, Bunegin I, Dujovny M, Hellstrom H, Jannetta PJ. Evoked potential changes during brain retraction in dogs. Stroke 1977;8:487–92.

19. Yamagata S, Carter LP, Erspamer RJ. Cortical ischemia: effect upon direct cortical response. Stroke 1982;13:9.

20. Sohmer H, Gafni M, Chisin R. Auditory nerve brain stem potentials in man and cat under hypoxic and hypercapnic conditions. Electroencephalogr Clin Neurophysiol 1982;53:506–12.

21. Sohmer H, Gafni M, Goitein K, Fainmesser P. Auditory nerve-brain stem evoked potentials in cats during manipulation of the cerebral perfusion pressure. Electroencephalogr Clin Neurophysiol 1983;55:198–202.

22. Sohmer H, Gafni M, Havatselet G. Persistence of auditory nerve response in severe cerebral ischemia. Electroencephalogr Clin Neurophysiol 1984;58:65–72.

23. Sundt TM, Sharbrough FW, Piepgras DG, Kearns TP, Messick JM, O'Fallon WM. Correlation of cerebral blood flow and electroencephalographic changes during carotid endarterectomy—with results of surgery and hemodynamics of cerebral ischemia. Mayo Clin Proc 1981;56:533–43.

24. Astrup J. Energy-requiring cell functions in the ischemic brain. Their critical supply and possible inhibition in protective therapy. J Neurosurg 1982;56:482–97.

25. Astrup J, Symon L, Branston NM, Lassen NA. Cortical evoked potential and extracellular K^+ and H^+ at critical levels of brain ischemia. Stroke 1977;8:51–57.

26. Hume AL, Cant BR. Conduction time in central somatosensory pathways in man. Electroencephalogr Clin Neurophysiol 1978;45:361–75.
27. Sutton LM, Frewen T, Marsh R, Jaggi J, Bruce DA. The effects of deep barbiturate coma on multimodality evoked potentials. J Neurosurg 1982;57:178–85.
28. Anderson DC, Bundlie S, Rockswold GL. Multimodality evoked potentials in closed head trauma. Arch Neurol 1984;41:369–74.
29. Rosenberg C, Wogensen K, Starr A. Auditory brainstem and middle-and long-latency evoked potentials in coma. Arch Neurol 1984;41:835–38.
30. Hall JW III, Huangfu M, Gennarelli TA. Auditory function in acute severe head injury. Laryngoscope 1982;92:883–90.
31. Nagao S, Roccaforte P, Moody RA. Acute intracranial hypertension and auditory brain-stem response. Part 1: changes in the auditory brain-stem and somatosensory evoked responses in intracranial hypertension in cats. J Neurosurg 1979;51:669–76.
32. Nagao S, Sunami N, Tsutsui T, Honma Y, Doi A, Nishimoto A. Serial observation of brain stem function by auditory brain stem responses in central transtentorial herniation. Surg Neurol 1982;17:355–57.
33. Starr A. Auditory brainstem responses in brain death. Brain 1976;99:543–54.
34. Tsubokawa T, Nichimoto H, Yamamoto T, Kitamura, M, Katayama, Y, Moriyasu, N. Assessment of brainstsem damage by the auditory brainstem response in acute severe head injury. J Neurol Neurosurg Psychiat 1980;43:1005–11.
35. Uziel A, Benezech J. Auditory brainstem response in comatose patients. Relationship with brainstem response and level of coma. Electroencephalogr Clin Neurophysiol 1978;45:515–24.

Chapter 10

Sensory Evoked Responses in the Diagnosis of Brain Death

James W. Hall III
Judy R. Mackey-Hargadine

A diagnosis of brain death requires evidence of irreversible destruction (or dysfunction) of neurons in the brain stem and cerebrum [1]. Cerebral death, without brain stem inactivity, is not equivalent to brain death. Numerous sets of criteria for definition of brain death have evolved, and are currently used in the United States and abroad [1,2]. Most sets of criteria employed for brain death require clinical evidence of apnea, cerebral nonresponsiveness, and absence of brain stem reflexes, with confirmation of CNS (central nervous system) inactivity from ancillary tests such as electroencephalogram (EEG) or cerebral blood flow (CBF) studies [1–6].

However, these ancillary tests are not clinically feasible in all cases. For example, bedside CBF study is not a commonly available clinical procedure. The clinical neurologic examination and EEG are not valid measures of brain integrity in patients who are drug intoxicated or receiving therapeutic paralyzing agents or CNS depressants [7]. Furthermore, valid measurement of the EEG in an intensive care unit (ICU) setting is compromised by serious technical problems [8–10] and, at best, provides information only on cerebral functional status [11,12]. Since the interpretation of the EEG requires a specially trained neurologist, a report of the results is not available immediately following testing. The resulting delay in the declaration of death can contribute to emotional and financial costs for the patient's family. Therefore, a clinical need exists for an electrophysiologic measure of CNS status that is not influenced by barbiturates or muscle paralyzers and that can be carried out at bedside, with immediate interpretation of findings.

Sensory evoked responses (SERs) are a potentially useful clinical technique for the evaluation of brain death [1,13,14]. There are at least four reasons why the auditory brain stem response (ABR) and short-latency somatosensory evoked response (SSER) are well suited for this important application. First, it is possible to make reliable and valid recordings of these responses in an ICU setting and to interpret the results promptly at bedside [15–18]. Second, these techniques are noninvasive and pose no risk to the patient, thus facilitating serial measurements. Third, both are electrophysiologic measures of brain stem and sensory cortical function, thus complementing the clinical neurologic examination and other cerebral electrophysiologic indexes such as the EEG and longer-latency SERs. Finally, neither of these SERs is seriously influenced by CNS depressants, including therapeutic, high dose barbiturates [15,16,19,20]. For these reasons, SERs may offer a clinically feasible and useful technique for confirming irreversible CNS dysfunction, particularly in patients with major complicating conditions such as drug and/or metabolic intoxication that preclude reliable assessment of brain stem and cerebral function by the clinical examination [6]. In this chapter, we review the literature on SERs in determination of brain death. We then present original data documenting the clinical utility of auditory AERs and SSERs in the documentation of CNS functional status, including the diagnosis of brain death.

REVIEW OF LITERATURE

There are two published studies of both auditory brain stem ABR and short-latency SSERs in brain death [13,21]. Goldie and colleagues measured SERs in two groups of patients with varied etiologies of brain injury [13]. Thirty-five patients, prior to SER assessment, had shown no clinical evidence of CNS function for several hours, an isoelectric EEG, and lack of spontaneous respiration—a clinical diagnosis of brain death. The other group consisted of fifty-three comatose patients with acute brain injury but some evidence of brain stem and cerebral functioning. Over three-fourths (77%) of the thirty-five brain dead patients had no ABR, including no wave I (eighth cranial nerve) component, whereas 16% of fifty patients with CNS function also yielded this pattern. A normal ABR was recorded in 52% of this latter group but never in the brain dead patients. Twenty-nine brain dead patients underwent SSER testing. All had a reliable Erb's point (brachial plexus) potential N_9, and in 69% a second wave complex in the 13 to 15 msec region (presumed to arise from the dorsal column nuclei and/or cervicomedullary junction) was observed. Absence of this wave complex was associated with cervical spinal cord transection. None of the brain dead patients showed an N_{20} (negative wave at 20 msec, presumably arising from thalamic/primary somatosensory cortical regions).

In the other brain-injured group, all patients yielded an Erb's point component and cervical spinal cord waves (13 to 15 msec wave components), and the majority (64%) showed at least unilateral evidence of N_{20}. Excessive electrical artifact precluded valid interpretation of five ABR recordings and one SSER recording. Goldie and colleagues concluded that both modalities of SERs can be useful in describing brain death and, in particular, that the absence of an ABR and the SSER beyond Erb's point is only seen in brain death [13]. They correctly noted, however, that the absence of any ABR components (wave I included) is an equivocal finding since it can result purely from peripheral otologic abnormality rather than CNS pathology. Therefore, their data suggested that the ABR may have somewhat limited value in this clinical application.

Consistent with the outcome of the study by Goldie and colleagues [13] were the findings of the French investigators Mauguière et al [21]. ABRs, SSERs, and EEG activity were measured in twenty comatose patients; thirteen with head injuries, six with vascular insults, and one with anoxia. In patients with absent brain stem reflexes and an isoelectric EEG (a total of eight) but not necessarily meeting clinical criteria for brain death, there were varied AB patterns, ranging from apparently normal waveforms to no response. SSERs in this group were characterized by a reliable wave complex in the 14 to 15 msec region yet no apparent N_{20} wave bilaterally. In another group consisting of seven clinically brain dead patients, an ABR wave I was recorded in two, and there was no ABR in the others. The SSER wave N_{14} (attributed to cervical generators) was consistently observed, a P_{15} wave was apparent in four cases, and none of the patients yielded an N_{20} component.

Starr, in the first clinical report on the use of the ABR in determination of brain death, described two characteristic outcomes in a series of twenty-seven patients with varied types of brain injuries including anoxia, trauma, and hemorrhage [22]. All met the following criteria for brain death: (1) no spontaneous respiration by visual inspection; (2) absence of motor responses to tactile, painful, visual, or auditory stimulation and absence of motor posturing; (3) no brain stem reflexes or cranial nerve function by examination; and (4) an isoelectric EEG. In this series, 41% showed an ABR wave I only, and in the remainder (59%) there was no response. Subsequent investigations have confirmed and expanded on Starr's observations [15,16,23–31]. Mjoen and colleagues, however, contend that "integrity of wave I and loss of other waves indicates activity in intracranial structures and, therefore, is inconsistent with the diagnosis of brain death" [28, p. 137]. Perhaps, as also suggested by Goldie et al in a discussion of the variable preservation of the SSER early (13 to 14 msec) wave complex in brain death, the ABR wave I absence or presence is associated with whether or not there is intracranial circulation [13]. We will demonstrate shortly, with group data correlating the ABR with nuclear CBF that both ABR outcomes are compatible with brain death. We also present evidence in support of Klug's claim that serial ABR recordings in patients neurologically decompensating can be useful in determining the most effective time for the application of sophisticated confirmatory procedures, like nuclear radiography, and in estimating the moment of CNS death [31].

SSER measurement, without the ABR was also reported in brain death.

Anziska and Cracco [32] recorded SSERs to median nerve stimulation in eleven patients meeting clinical criteria for brain death, as described for the study by Goldie et al [13]. It is important to note that patients with drug overdose and hypothermia were excluded. All the patients showed a peripheral N_9 potential. In agreement with Goldie et al, 64% of the group (seven of eleven) also had a reliable wave complex in the 13 to 15 msec latency region. The authors presume that these components arise from the cervical spinal cord, medullary brain stem, and perhaps more rostral brain stem structures. One patient unexpectedly consistently showed an N_{20} (thalamic/cortical) component on four separate SSER test sessions, even though there was apparently no cerebral circulation by arteriography. In the remainder of the group, there was no evidence of the SSER component, and longer-latency components were not recorded from any patients.

Another report, allegedly on the topic of SSERs in brain death, did not present data or specific clinical experiences [33]. Twenty-two brain-injured patients were studied with SSERs; however, only three were mechanically ventilated at the time of testing, and only two yielded an isoelectric EEG. None apparently met definite clinical criteria for brain death. Also, Rumpl and colleagues in a study of SSERs in twenty-three comatose patients, found no N_{20} wave in six who were brain dead as confirmed by an isoelectric EEG [34]. Each of the six showed a wave complex in the 13 to 15 msec region.

In summary, then, ABR findings in brain death are rather straightforward; namely, there is a wave I component with no later waves or no response including absence of wave I. In both cases, evidence of brain stem integrity is lacking. SSER outcome in brain death, in contrast, appears to be more variable. The peripheral (Erb's point) component is a constant feature, but later wave components may or may not be observed. A wave complex in the 13 to 15 msec region is reportedly observed in approximately two out of three clinically brain dead patients. This poses a dilemma in SSER interpretation; that is, if this wave component is not recorded, there is a substantial likelihood of cervical spinal injury [13], and therefore, the SSER is not a valid measure of more rostral CNS status. Conversely, the presence of this wave complex, later-latency components of which may reflect brain stem and diencephalic neuronal activity [32–39], would seem to be incompatible with a definition of irreversible brain stem destruction or dysfunction. At least five factors contribute to the confusion regarding SSER patterns in brain death, including differences among studies in the postinjury time of assessment, the criteria for brain death, recording techniques (especially electrode arrays), and a poor understanding of the neural generators of the wave components and the nature of blood supply (intra- versus extracranial) in the cervico-medullary-pontine region of the CNS. Most perplexing and disconcerting is the reported case of a preserved N_{20} wave component in a clinically brain dead patient [32] because researchers agree that the N_{20} wave arises from at least thalamic [36], if not primary cortical, regions [32,33,38–43].

CLINICAL EXPERIENCE

Methods

In a 12 mo period we carried out over 250 ABR and 30 SSER assessments in acute, severely head-injured patients. All testing was done at bedside in a surgical intensive care unit (SICU) with commercially available instrumentation. The initial assessment was conducted within 24 hr postinjury in three-fourths (74%) of the group. The majority of patients was chemically paralyzed and/or managed with high dose barbiturates. In approximately one-third of the series, SERs were used in the determination of brain death, usually in conjunction with nuclear CBF studies.

ABR assessment was carried out with a Nicolet CA-1000/DC-2000 evoked potential system according to the following protocol. Acoustic stimuli were clicks of 0.1 msec duration presented at a rate of 21.1/sec and at an intensity level of 85 to 95 dB (normal click hearing level) with TDH-39 earphones and MX-41/AR cushions enclosed within aural domes and coupled to circumaural cushions. Stimuli were always presented monaurally to the right and left ears. The ABR was detected with gold cup electrodes. The positive voltage electrode was at a high forehead, midline location, the negative voltage (earclip) electrode was on the stimulated ear, and the ground electrode was at a low forehead location. In addition to this standard electrode array, simultaneous four-channel ABR recordings were made with all patients in an attempt to clarify waveform morphology [18]. The neural signal was amplified (x 100,000) and filtered at 30 to 3,000 Hz, whenever possible, or 150 to 3,000 Hz if low frequency artifact was present. A minimum of 512 sample points was used. Interelectrode impedance was always less than 5,000 ohm. ABR data were analyzed and interpreted by the first author (JWH) without knowledge of CBF outcome.

SSERs were stimulated and averaged with a Neurotrac (Interspec) instrument. Stimuli were 1,000 electrical pulses of 0.1 msec duration delivered to the median nerve of each arm at a rate of 4.1/sec. Neural activity was detected with a dual-channel, subcutaneous needle electrode (Grass) recording array. One channel employed a negative voltage electrode over the stimulus ipsilateral Erb's point (supraclavicular) and a positive voltage forehead electrode. With the second channel, the negative voltage electrode was located over the parietal cortex contralateral to the stimulated side, and the positive voltage electrode was on the forehead. A large, disk-type ground electrode was placed on the proximal forearm on the stimulated side. Neural activity was amplified (x 100,000) and band-pass filtered (5 to 1,500 Hz) before the averaging process. Interelectrode impedance was always less than 5,000 ohm. SSER data were interpreted by the second author (JMH).

CBF measurements were made at bedside within 12 hr of the ABR assessment with a mobile system (Ohio Nuclear, Sigma 420). Following the intravenous administration of approximately 20 mc of technetium, serial anterior flow images and immediate and delayed static images of the head were obtained. Nuclear CBF data were interpreted by nuclear radiology staff without knowledge of ABR outcome.

Group Data

Auditory Brain Stem Response and Cerebral Blood Flow

As displayed in Table 10.1, there is a strong association between the ABR and CBF outcome. Data are displayed for a total of eighty combined studies in sixty-one patients. In our experience, normal ABR has invariably been associated with a nuclear CBF study demonstrating flow. We have also often recorded an ABR with abnormal brain stem transmission times (prolonged caudal or rostral brain stem latency intervals) in patients with evidence of a nuclear CBF study demonstrating flow. All but two patients in this series with only an ABR wave I or no response showed no evidence of nuclear CBF. Since in each of these exceptions the CBF measurement preceded ABR recording by more than 6 hr, we cannot rule out a change in pathophysiologic status from one study to the next. It is important to point out that 70% of the patients with no response at the time of joint ABR/CBF evaluation had demonstrated a reliable ABR or at least a wave I component on previous assessments, thus effectively ruling out serious peripheral otologic abnormality. Statistical analysis indicates that ABR and CBF outcome are significantly correlated (chi-square, $p < .00001$).

SER Patterns in Suspected Brain Death

Patterns of SER outcome found in patients neurologically unresponsive and undergoing assessment in the determination of brain death were varied, ranging

Table 10.1 Correlation of Eighty ABR and Nuclear CBF Studies in Sixty-one Brain-injured Patients

	ABR			
CBF	*Normal*	*Abnormal*[a]	*Wave I Only*	*No Response*
Normal	17	14	1	0
Asymmetric/delayed	0	1	1	0
None	0	3	17	26[b]

Note: Correlation significant at $p < .001$ (chi-square = 66.7213, degrees of freedom = 6).

In patients with ABR asymmetry, data are from the least involved side.

[a]Abnormal wave I to III and/or III to V latency prolongation or absent wave V.

[b]Eighteen patients in this category (70%) showed an ABR on initial assessment. Eight patients had no ABR on initial assessment.

from apparently normal responses to the absence of any SER, including no peripheral component (ABR). We stress that the patients in our series did not necessarily meet all clinical criteria for brain death. In particular, respiratory (apnea) reflexes were not consistently evaluated. Evaluations for brain death were initiated on the basis of severe neurologic decompensation and/or evidence of an apparently fatal injury by CT, particularly evidence of transtentorial herniation or physiologic abnormalitaies [eg., grossly elevated intracranial pressure (ICP), hypoxia, hypotension].

As suggested by the data in Table 10.1, some patients in our series yielded unequivocally normal SERs. The normal ABR was characterized by well-formed and reliable wave components I, III, and V, with all brain stem transmission times within normal limits. The normal SSER was characterized by a distinct Erb's point component and a distinct 13 to 15 msec wave complex and N_{20}. Of the patients showing a normal SER, approximately one-half were treated with chemical paralyzing agents or barbiturates, rendering the neurologic exam invalid. Average blood level at assessment was 35 μg/ml. A normal or even abnormal, but reliably recorded, ABR and/or SSER was considered unequivocal evidence of CNS functioning and, therefore, was not compatible with brain death. The most distinctive and clear-cut finding consistent with brain death was a reliable peripheral response component—that is, an ABR wave I or an SSER Erb's point component—and usually the 13 to 15 msec wave complex and no subsequent SER components. Less than 10% of the patients in this series had no peripheral component on ABR testing, and none of the patients showed no peripheral component bilaterally on SSER assessment. To record SSER subcutaneous needle electrodes were routinely used. We have previously described SER patterns found in patients evaluated for brain death in more detail elsewhere [15,16].

CASE REPORTS

Case 1: ABR and CBF

The patient was a 24-year-old male who sustained a gunshot wound to the right temporal region, with no exit. He was first taken to an outlying hospital where physical examination showed a small pupil on the right that was reactive to light; a large, unreactive left pupil; and spontaneous movement of the upper extremities. Hypotension was never noted. He was intubated and given mannitol intravenously and diazepam.

Within 45 min after the injury, the patient was transferred via Life Flight helicopter to the Hermann Hospital. At the time of neurosurgery consultation, (1.5 hr postinjury), both pupils were fixed and dilated, there was spontaneous movement of all four extremities to deep painful stimulation, and Glasgow Coma Scale (GCS) score was 7. Emergency medical therapy included dexamethasone and mannitol. Alcohol blood level at admission was 158 mg/dl.

Skull X-ray revealed a linear fracture from the right temporal to parietal-occipital regions. Computed tomography (CT) also showed the skull fracture, plus a right subdural hematoma and fragments in the right parietal-occipital area. The patient was taken to the operating room for debridement of the wound and placement of an ICP monitor and then to the SICU.

Initial auditory evoked response AER assessment was carried out in the SICU at 14 hr postinjury. At the time of testing, mean arterial pressure (MAP) was 83 mm Hg, ICP was 25 mm Hg (cerebral perfusion pressure, CPP, of 58 mm Hg), arterial blood gases were adequate (PaO$_2$ of over 200 mm Hg, PaCO$_2$ of 21 mm Hg) and body temperature was normal (37°C). Medications included morphine, metacurine, and mannitol. Neurologic examination 2 hr after administration of the muscle paralysis agent showed pupils fixed in midposition, no movement to pain (flaccid), and absence of corneal, gag, and oculocephalic (doll's eyes) reflexes. The residual influence of medication on neurologic findings could not be ruled out. As illustrated in Figure 10.1, left ear acoustic stimulation produced a well-formed ABR, with all major components clearly observed and brain stem transmission time (4.38 msec) within normal limits. There was no auditory middle-latency response (AMR) with left ear stimulation. There was also no ABR or AMR with right ear stimulation at the maximum intensity level, (95 dB hearing level) consistent with the aforementioned radiographic evidence of right temporal bone fracture.

Thirty-one hours postinjury, AER measurement was repeated. At the time of this assessment, MAP was 73 mm Hg (maintained with dopamine), ICP was 17 mm Hg (CPP of 56 mm Hg), temperature remained normal (37.5°C)

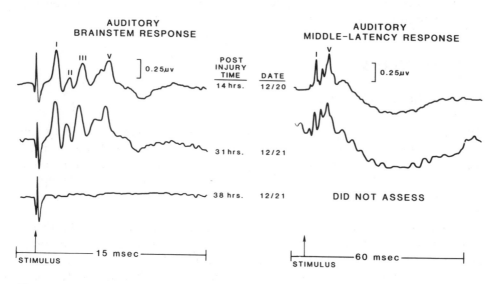

Figure 10.1   Serial AER recordings for a 24-yr-old with a severe head injury (Case 1).

and arterial blood gases were good (PaO_2 of 218 mm Hg, $PaCO_2$ of 30.2 mm Hg). Medical therapy consisted of morphine and metacurine. A neurologic examination within the previous hour, following reversal of muscle paralysis, revealed pupils that were 3 mm and nonreactive bilaterally, no movement to deep pain, and absence of the previously noted brain stem reflexes. Again, there was a normal and reliably recorded ABR, but no AMR, with left ear stimulation, and no responses to right ear stimulation (see left side of Figure 10.1). Nuclear CBF study within 30 min after the evoked response testing showed evidence of bilateral cerebral perfusion (Figure 10.2). Even with apparent reversal of metacurine, the chronic drug use may have influenced the neurologic examination, and clinical findings, therefore, could not be confidently used in the declaration of brain death.

The third and final AER assessment was carried out later on postinjury day 1 (at 38 hr). At the time, MAP was 80 mm Hg (dopamine maintained), ICP was 50 mm Hg (CPP of 30 mm Hg), temperature was 39.4°C, and arterial blood gases were comparable to earlier values (PaO_2 of 217 mm Hg, $PaCO_2$ of 24 mm Hg). Medical therapy had been discontinued. Neurologic examination findings were unchanged. As shown in Figure 10.1, there was no ABR bilaterally. A follow-up nuclear CBF study early the next day (postinjury day 2) produced no evidence of perfusion in the region of the anterior or middle

24, male, GSW

Study 1
(12/21)

Study 2
(12/22)

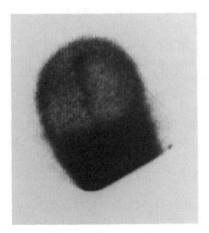
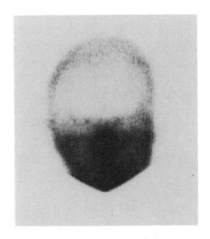

Figure 10.2   Serial nuclear CBF (perfusion) findings for a 24-yr-old male with a severe head injury (Case 1).

cerebral arteries or the superior sagittal sinus. In light of the physical examination findings and absence of cerebral circulation, the patient was declared dead at 56 hr postinjury. He was then taken to the operating room for a donor nephrectomy and splenectomy.

Comment

This case illustrates at least four main points:

1. Serial AER data can be reliably obtained in an ICU, beginning within hours of severe traumatic head injury.
2. Trauma in the temporal bone region may preclude ABR measurement. However, bilaterally absent responses secondary to head injury are unusual at the initial assessment (typically, completed within 48 hr postinjury), occurring in less than 5% of our series of over 200 patients.
3. A normal ABR can be recorded in patients neurologically unresponsive.
4. ABR and nuclear CBF outcome are correlated in severe head injury and can contribute to prompt, complete, and most important, accurate declaration of brain death and, therefore, facilitate successful donation of organs.

Case 2: ABR in Barbiturate Coma

The patient was a 19-year-old male involved in a motor vehicle accident at 2 A.M. in a town approximately 75 mi from Houston. At the scene he reportedly had temporary loss of consciousness for an undetermined length of time but subsequently was moving all extremities and was appropriate on neurologic testing. He was never hypotensive.

The patient was transported to Hermann Hospital via Life Flight helicopter. Upon arrival, physical examination revealed stable vital signs, two fractured ribs on the right, dislocation of the right hip, and possible mandibular fracture. Neurologically, pupils were 3 mm and sluggishly reactive to light bilaterally, and the patient was alert and oriented, with motor and sensory function intact and a GCS of 15. The patient was well oxygenated and hyperventilated (PaO_2, 143 mm Hg; $PaCO_2$, 26 mm Hg). Skull films were negative. The patient had difficulty maintaining an airway in the emergency center and, therefore, was nasally intubated. CT showed fracture of the lateral wall of the left maxillary antrum associated with hemorrhage but no definite brain lesion or gross hematoma. He was admitted for evaluation of facial and orthopedic injuries.

At 16 hr postinjury (in the evening), the patient was taken to the operating room for maxillofacial repairs. Surgery was uneventful, but postoperatively in the recovery room he arrested, developed laryngospasm, and was difficult to re-intubate. Lowest heart rate was 30/min and blood pressure was not palpable momentarily. The patient was resuscitated, and 3 hr after surgery, when transferred to the SICU, he was following commands, moving purposefully, and breathing spontaneously. Neurosurgical consultation was requested 2 hr later following respiratory/cardiovascular instability and neurologic deterioration. Pupils were 2 mm and reacted sluggishly bilaterally, and the corneal reflex was also sluggish. There was a cough reflex and GCS was 5 (E_2, M_2, V_1). A second CT scan showed no definitive intracranial hematoma, a normal-appearing ventricular system, and well-visualized basal cisterns.

Physiologic and neurologic status during the patient's 20 day hospital course are summarized and correlated with ABR findings in Table 10.2. Initially neurologic status improved (GCS to 8) and the ABR was normal bilaterally. However, a third CT scan on postinjury day 4 showed the development of diffuse cerebral edema since the previous scan and a possible small area of hemorrhagic contusion in the right posterior temporal area. Ventricles were smaller and the perimesencephalic cistern was not apparent. A rostral ABR latency abnormality was observed bilaterally.

Repeated elevations of ICP (to 37 mm Hg) required hyperosmolar (mannitol) therapy, and by the ninth postinjury day, serum osmolarity was in the high 200s. The increased ICP was no longer responsive to mannitol, and barbiturate coma was initiated with a bolus of pentobarbital (300 mg IV). This produced only a mild reduction in ICP, and it was followed by a second bolus (700 mg IV), which reduced ICP to below 20 mm Hg. Barbiturate infusion was thereafter continued in an attempt to maintain ICP below 20 mm Hg. The previously recorded rostral ABR abnormalities reversed. The ABR was again well within normal limits bilaterally. This therapeutic approach was effective until the eleventh postinjury day, when further elevation in ICP demanded more aggressive barbiturate therapy. As indicated in Table 10.2, barbiturate blood levels subsequently increased to a high of 78 μg/ml. On postinjury days 12 through 15, abnormally prolonged rostral brain stem transmission times were again repeatedly recorded (see Table 10.2).

A third CT scan was attempted on the fifteenth day postinjury but was aborted when the pupils became dilated bilaterally at the start of the scanning. The patient was immediately returned to the SICU. Hyperventilation and an additional bolus of mannitol failed to reverse the pupillary abnormalities. However, the ABR abnormalities were again reversed at the 6 P.M. test session.

During the next 5 day (postinjury days 16 through 20), barbiturate blood levels remained above 50 μg/ml, and consequently, neurologic status appeared unchanged by clinical examination (dilated, unreactive pupils; absent brain stem reflexes; GCS of 3). ICP, unfortunately, was persistently elevated (greater than 30 mm Hg) during the intervals between AER tests with transient plateaus in the 40 to 50 mm Hg range despite maximal, previously effective, therapy. Through postinjury day 16, there continued to be rostral ABR abnormalities. Two days later, caudal brain stem transmission time also became prolonged. On the morning of the twentieth postinjury day, there was no ABR bilaterally. Based on this evidence of CNS inactivity, nuclear CBF studies were requested. They showed absence of blood flow in middle and cerebral artery regions and

Table 10.2   Chronologic Summary of Neurologic and ABR Findings in a 19-yr-old Male with Acute Brain Injury

		Test Session/(Postinjury Day)					
Parameter	*Test Day*	*1* / *1*	*2* / *4*	*3* / *5*	*4* / *6*	*5* / *8*	*6* / *9*
Barbiturates (μg/ml)		—	—	—	—	—	—
Temperature (°C)		37.7	37.2	37.5	37.7	37.7	38.1
ICP (mm Hg)		NA	NA	31	19	13	9
Glasgow Coma Scale score		5	8	7	5	6	3
Pupils (reactivity/ size, mm)[a]		+/3	+/3	+/3	+/3	+/3	+/4
ABR (latency)							
Rostral		+	+	+/−	+/−	+/−	+
Caudal		+	+	+	+	+	+

[a] + = Normal; +/− = Abnormal; − = No response.
[b] Nuclear cerebral angiography showed no CBF, compatible with brain death; CPP = 37 mm Hg at the time of testing.

no superior sagittal sinus flow. Following discussions with the family, it was decided to maintain cardiopulmonary function if possible, although hypotension and diabetes insipidus were now apparent. The next day the patient was declared brain dead.

Comment

Serial SER recordings are particularly useful in documenting the neurologic status of head-injured patients in deep barbiturate coma and may play an important role in management. In this illustrative case, information from ABR assessments initially complemented neurologic findings and monitored physiologic parameters. From day 15 onward, however, barbiturate blood levels were high, and as a consequence, brain stem reflexes, including the pupillary response, were not detectable and the ABR provided essentially the single index of CNS integrity. On two occasions, ABR abnormalities following elevated ICP were clearly reversed with aggressive medical therapy. The development of caudal, as well as previously recorded rostral, ABR abnormalities on the eighteenth postinjury day provided early evidence of impending, end-stage CNS decompensation in the absence of valid clinical neurologic signs. A rostral-to-caudal progression on ABR abnormalities associated with increased ICP (and decreased CPP) has been documented previously [15,16]. This sequence culminated with the finding of no ABR on the twentieth day (twenty-fifth ABR test session), which led to an additional confirmatory test (nuclear CBF) and a rational basis for counseling the family regarding brain death.

		13 15 (9 A.M.)	14 15 (6 P.M.)			21 18 (7 A.M.)	22 18 (3 P.M.)		
9 11	10 12			17 16	19 17			24 19	25 20
2	10	20	35	78	66	70	76	74	50
37.2	36.1	37.5	37.7	38.3	37.7	38.3	36.6	37.2	36.9
9	18	9	11	31	10	29	6	26	29[b]
3	3	3	3	3	3	3	3	3	3
+/6	±/2	−/6	−/6	−/5	−/5	−/6	−/6	−/6	−/6
+	+/−	+/−	+	+/−	+/−	+/−	+/−	+	−
+	+	+	+	+	+	+	+/−	+/−	−

Case 3: Serial SSERs and Compressed Spectral Array EEG

A 30-yr-old male was involved in a motor vehicle accident. Initial GCS was 4. Pupils were 6 mm on the right, 2 mm on the left, and nonreactive bilaterally. He was taken to the operating room for an ICP monitor. Opening pressure was 13 cm H_2O. Emergency CT showed a hemorrhagic contusion in the right temporal-frontal region and diffuse cerebral edema. ABRs and AMRs (cortical), initially measured within 12 hr post injury, were normal bilaterally. Throughout the first 8 days of the patient's hospital course, ICP was repeatedly elevated transiently but responded to hyperventilation and mannitol therapy. During this period, daily AER assessments occasionally showed evidence of normal brain stem and cortical functioning although significant peripheral (middle ear) otologic pathology confounded consistently confident interpretation of the recordings. Barbiturate therapy, which was begun on the ninth postinjury day for management of elevated ICP, suppressed the cortical components of the AMR.

Serial measurements of SSERs and compressed spectral array (CSA)-EEG were initiated on the tenth postinjury day to assess cerebral status electrophysiologically during the barbiturate coma [44–50]. These electrophysiologic data are correlated with physiologic parameters in Figure 10.3. On the first assessment, there was a well-formed and reliable SSER N_{20} wave (only waveforms for left median nerve stimulation are shown). Central conduction time (CCT), from the Erb's point component to N_{20} component, was 10.9 msec. The CSA-EEG was bilaterally symmetrical, with a spectral edge of 7 to 8 Hz. As displayed in the right portion of Figure 10.3, ICP was 20 mm Hg,

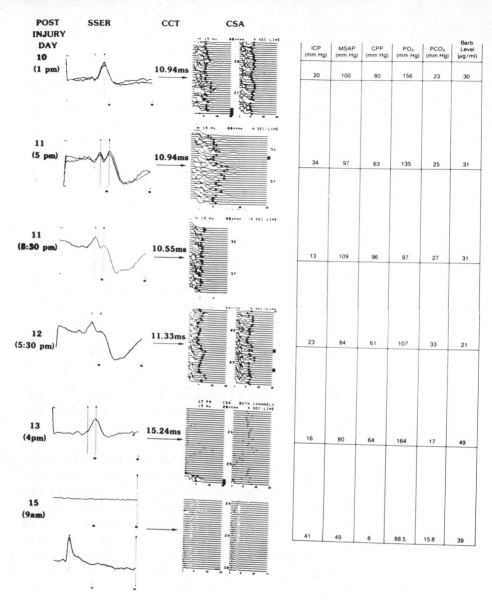

Figure 10.3 Serial SSER and CSA-EEG recordings for a 30-yr-old male with severe head injury. Electrophysiologic data are related to physiologic parameters (right side of figure).

CPP was 80 mm Hg, blood gases were adequate, and the barbiturate blood level was 30 μ/ml.

The following day, ICP had increased to 34 mm Hg and CPP decreased to 63 mm Hg. A bi-peaked SSER N_{20} wave was recorded, although CCT to the first peak was unchanged, and the CSA-EEG spectral edge was comparable to previous findings. Later on the eleventh postinjury day, ICP had been reduced (13 mm Hg) and CPP increased (96 mm Hg), with an apparently corresponding reduction in the SSER CCT (to 10.5 msec) and a less pronounced second peak in the N_{20} complex. CSA-EEG spectral edge was more restricted (5 Hz). Over the next 2 day, the SSER deteriorated. First (day 12), the CCT increased significantly (to 11.3 msec) as CPP decreased again (to 61 mm Hg). Also, $PaCO_2$ was substantially lower (17 mm Hg). Then (day 13, 5:30 P.M.) there was a further increase in CCT (to 15.2 msec). No CSA-EEG was recorded, but barbiturate blood level had increased to 49 μg/ml from 21 μg/ml on the previous day. Within 10 hrs, there was no SSER (a distinct peripheral component was still present) and no CSA-EEG activity. CPP was 8 mm Hg, and blood gases were abnormal. The patient subsequently showed no evidence of nuclear CBF.

Comment

The ABR provides information in brain stem function, and the AMR may be useful as one measure of cortical activity. As illustrated by this case, however, the SSER and CSA-EEG offer additional and clinically valuable documentation of CNS integrity [44–50]. In patients with serious acute or subacute peripheral otologic pathology, the AERs have limited application. Also, the apparent suppression of the AMR by relatively low barbiturate blood levels precludes the valid application of this auditory response in many patients [15,16]. In Case 3, the SSER showed distinctive abnormalities with reduction in CPP, even though the CSA-EEG appeared unchanged. These abnormalities were partially reversed with additional mannitol therapy but then became more pronounced with a second reduction in CPP. This is perhaps an example of the heightened vulnerability of the CNS with repeated insults, such as hypotension, hypoxia, or increased ICP, that we and others have observed with electrophysiologic monitoring [30,51]. The presence of distinct CSA-EEG activity in spite of barbiturate therapy suggested that the dose was therapeutically inadequate, despite blood levels in the low 30s (μg/ml). As in the other two case reports, SERs in Case 3 provided prompt indication of the most useful time for confirmation of brain death with nuclear CBF studies.

DISCUSSION

As stated in accepted guidelines for the determination of death, criteria should:

1. Eliminate errors in classifying a living individual as dead, 2. allow as few errors as possible in classifying a dead body as alive, 3. allow a determination to be

made without unreasonable delay, 4. be adaptable to a variety of clinical situations, and 5. be explicit and accessible to verification. [6, p. 2185]

Our clinical experience suggests that SERs fulfill these criteria. By completing the SER assessment as soon as possible post injury and by making statements on CNS status only when a distinct peripheral component has been recorded, the most serious type of error in the determination of brain death, a false positive error, is effectively eliminated; i.e., the absence of an SER, in the presence of a peripheral component, is invariably associated with irreversible cessation of CNS functioning. We have recorded reliable SERs in patients with apparently fatal injuries and with a neurologic examination that strongly suggested brain death. It is inconceivable, however, that a person with irreversible cessation of all functions of the entire brain, including the brain stem, could generate a reliable and repeatable SER.

There are a number of advantages to applying SERs in the determination of brain death. They can be recorded, noninvasively, within hours of the injury, in virtually any hospital environment, including the emergency room. They are not seriously influenced by intoxicants, barbiturates, or chemical paralyzing agents. They pose no risk to the patient, require 1 hr or less of test time, do not usually interfere with patient care, and are reasonably priced, relative to other diagnostic hospital procedures like CT. Unlike the EEG, SERs lend themselves to immediate and concise interpretation. A trained clinical neurophysiologist and/or audiologist, with experience in measuring evoked potentials in acute brain-injured patients, can generate a clinical report within minutes of the conclusion of testing. Response waveforms can be graphically displayed, labeled, and verified by other neurophysiologists and medical personnel. It is, perhaps, misleading to refer to SERs as objective measures of brain function since the interpretation of findings remains a subjective process. However, these electrophysiologic measurements do introduce standardization and verification to the clinical evaluation of neurologic functioning.

In a recent case report, Taylor and colleagues described serial ABR findings in a 33-mo-old with a severe hypoxic-ischemic insult following near drowning [52]. This account is noteworthy because the authors offer their findings as evidence that an ABR reappeared after it was not detected for several days and, therefore, may not be a valid measure of CNS status in determination of brain death. They stress that the patient at no time fulfilled criteria for brain death and conclude that "absent auditory brain-stem responses cannot be used in isolation as a criterion for brain death" (p. 1170). We do not take issue with this conclusion because it is unlikely that any single clinical procedure is infallible. We do, however, disagree with the authors' interpretation of their data that led to this conclusion. There is a fundamental principle in clinical ABR measurement: the validity of brain stem response data is assured only with confirmation of peripheral auditory system integrity. Taylor et al state, without any supporting data, that the loss of the ABR in their patient appeared to be secondary to brain stem damage rather than cochlear abnormality. What they do not discuss, regrettably, is the considerable likelihood that the disappearance of an ABR, including wave I, as measured on postinsult days 5 and 9, is due to middle ear pathology. The ABR waveforms that were reported for each of these test sessions showed blunted, irregular, and nondescript wave components. Furthermore, at the next assessment (day 14), the wave I component appeared markedly delayed. One might also take issue with their identification of waves II and III in the waveform recorded that day.

We have repeatedly observed a similar pattern of ABR changes in selected children and adults with severe brain injury who have remained comatose and mechanically ventilated for prolonged periods and have correlated disappearance and reappearance of an ABR with audiologically/otologically documented evolution and resolution of middle ear pathology [15,17]. In some cases, we have had to employ special stimulation or measurement techniques, such as bone conduction signals or multichannel recordings, to generate clinically useful data [18]. This is not to imply that reversal of brain stem component (waves III, IV, V) abnormalities is not possible since there are also examples of this phenomenon in the literature [15–17,51], and we have recently observed it in brain-injured infants. We emphasize, however, the importance of clinical documentation of peripheral auditory status prior to inference of brain stem dysfunction from an abnormal ABR and the confirmation of equivocal ABR findings with SSERs. Without such documentation, the conclusions of the study by Taylor and colleagues are suspect and should not be used as a basis for questioning the validity of the ABR in the determination of brain death [52].

As a result of the clinical advantages noted here, SERs can facilitate prompt determination of brain death and can clearly indicate the appropriate time for other confirmatory tests like nuclear CBF measurements. The elimination of an unreasonable delay in the determination of brain death is particularly important in major medical centers with active organ transplantation programs. Prompt determination of brain death also reduces the patient's hospital cost and emotional trauma for the patient's family.

The group data and case reports in this chapter support the following general conclusions. Application of SERs in determination of brain death is clinically feasible and useful, particularly when chemical paralysis and/or high dose barbiturate therapy invalidate the neurologic examination and other confirmatory measure like the EEG. The validity of SERs in the determination of brain death is confirmed by the strong association between these electrophysiologic measures and nuclear CBF. Previous clinical reports have suggested that the application of SERs in determining brain death might be compromised by a high occurrence rate of the equivocal finding of no response. This finding cannot be confidently used as evidence of CNS dysfunction because it may reflect, instead, serious peripheral sensory pathology. For example, Goldie et al found no ABR including the absence of a wave I component, in 77% of thirty-five patients evaluated for brain death [13]. Notably, however, their criteria for subject selection included lack of spontaneous respiration, no neurologic evidence of CNS function for several hours, and a previously isoelectric EEG. In our series, in contrast, only eight patients (less than 13%) showed no ABR on initial assessment. As illustrated by our case reports, the presence of reliable peripheral sensory components in most of our patients is probably a reflection of our ICU protocol—i.e., assessment as soon as possible following injury and then serial measurements thereafter. The approach is most useful in assuring the validity of SERs in the determination of brain death.

ACKNOWLEDGMENTS

E. Edmund Kim, M.D., Department of Radiology, University of Texas Medical School, provided and interpreted the nuclear CBF data reported in this chapter. Denice P. Brown, Ph.D., and Wende Yellin, M.S., Audiology Service, Hermann Hospital, and Chaudry Saleem, D.V.M., Division of Neurosurgery, University of Texas Medical School, assisted in SER data collection. Jason Charles Hall contributed to the literature review. Interspec Incorporated, Conshohocken, Pennsylvania, supplied the Neurotrac instrumentation used in CSA-EEG recordings and most SSER measurements.

Portions of this chapter were presented at the Annual Meeting of the American Association of Neurological Surgeons in San Francisco, April 9–11, 1984.

REFERENCES

1. Korein J. Brain death. In: Kottrel JE, Turndorf H, eds. Anesthesiology in neurosurgery. St. Louis: C.V. Mosby, 1980;282–31.
2. Korein J, ed. Brain death: interrelated medical and social issues. Ann NY Acad Sci 1978;315:1–433.
3. Jennett B, Gleave J, Wilson P. Brain death in three neurosurgical units. Brit J Med 1981;282:533–39.
4. Ingvar DH, Widen L. Brain death; summary of a symposium. Lakartidningen 1972;34:3804–14.
5. An appraisal of the criteria of cerebral death; a summary statement: a collaborative study sponsored by the National Institute of Neurological Diseases and Stroke (Contract N01-NS-1-2316) JAMA 1977;237:982–86.
6. Guidelines for the determination of death. Report of the medical consultants on the diagnosis of death to the president's commission for the study of ethical problems in medicine and biomedical and behavioral research. JAMA 1981;246:2184–86.
7. Plum F, Posner JB. The diagnosis of stupor and coma, 3rd ed. Philadelphia: F.A. Davis, 1980.
8. Grossman RJ. Electrophysiologic evaluation of the central nervous system after trauma. In: Odom GL, ed. Central nervous system trauma. Bethesda, Md.: Research Study Report, NIH, NINCDS, 1979;159–76.
9. Bickford RG. The values and limitations of EEG monitoring in intensive care units. Electroencephalogr Clin Neurophysiol 1972;32:101.

10. Burgess R, Cant BR, Hume AL, Priestley LC, Shaw NA. Cerebral monitoring by compressed spectral array. New Zealand Med J 1977;86:521–23.
11. Bennett D. The EEG in determination of brain death. In: Korein J, ed. Brain death; interrelated medical and social issues. Ann NY Acad Sci 1978;315:110–20.
12. Hughes J. Limitations of the EEG in the diagnosis of brain death. In: Korein J, ed. Brain death; interrelated medical and social issues. Ann NY Acad Sci 1978;315:121–36.
13. Goldie WD, Chiappa KH, Young RR, Brooks EB. Brainstem auditory and short-latency somatosensory evoked responses in brain death. Neurology 1981;31:248–56.
14. Trojaborg W, Jorgensen EO. Evoked cortical potentials in patients with "isoelectric" EEG's. Electroencephalogr Clin Neurophysiol 1973;35:301–05.
15. Hall JW III, Mackey-Hargadine J. Auditory evoked responses in severe head injury. Seminars in Hearing 1984;5:313–16.
16. Hall JW III, Mackey-Hargadine J, Allen SJ. Monitoring neurologic status of comatose patients in the intensive care unit. In Jacobson JJ, ed. Auditory brainstem response audiometry. San Diego: College Hill Press, 1985;253–83.
17. Hall JW III, Huangfu M, Gennarelli TA, Dolinskas CA, Olsen K, Berry GA. Auditory evoked responses, impedance measures and diagnostic speech audiometry in severe head injury. Otolaryngol Head Neck Surg 1983;91:50–60.
18. Hall JW III, Morgan SH, Mackey-Hargadine J, Aguilar EA III, Jahrsdoerfer RA. Neuro-otologic applications of simultaneous multi-channel auditory evoked response recordings. Laryngoscope 1984;94:883–89.
19. Sutton LM, Frewen T, Marsh R, Jaggi J, Bruce DA. The effects of deep barbiturate coma on multimodality evoked potentials. J Neurosurg 1982;57:178–85.
20. Newlon PG, Greenberg RP, Enas GG, Becker DP. Effects of therapeutic pentobarbital coma on multimodality evoked potentials recorded from severely head-injured patients. Neurosurgery 1983;12:613–19.
21. Mauguière F, Grand C, Fischer C, Courjon J. Aspects des potentials évoqués auditifs et somesthésiques précoces dans les comas neurologiques et la mort cérébrale. Rev EEG Neurophysiol 1982;12:280–86.
22. Starr A. Auditory brain-stem responses in brain death. Brain 1976;99:543–54.
23. Tsubokawa T, Nichimoto H, Yamamoto T, Kitamura M, Katayama Y, Moriyasu N. Assessment of brainstem damage by the auditory brainstem response in acute severe head injury. J Neurol Neurosurg Psychiat 1980;43:1005–11.
24. Seales DM, Rossiter BS, Weinstein ME. Brainstem auditory evoked responses in patients comatose as a result of blunt head trauma. J Trauma 1979;19:347–53.
25. Greenberg RP, Becker DP, Miller JD, Mayer DJ. Evaluation of brain function in severe head trauma with multimodality evoked potentials. Part II. Localization of brain dysfunction in correlation with post-traumatic neurologic condition. J Neurosurg 1977;47:163–77.
26. Lütschg J, Pfenninger J, Ludin HP, Fassela F. Brain-stem auditory evoked potentials and early somatosensory evoked potentials in neurointensively treated comatose children. Am J Dis Child 1983;137:421–26.
27. Yagi T, Baba N. Evaluation of the brain-stem function by the auditory brain-stem response and the caloric vestibular reaction in comatose patients. Arch Otolaryngol 1983;238:33–43.
28. Mjoen S, Nordby HC, Torvic A. Auditory evoked brainstem responses (ABR) in coma due to severe head trauma. Acta Otolaryngol 1983;95:131–38.

29. Kallwellis G, Roder H, Rabending G. Auditory evoked brain stem potentials in patients in coma and brain death. Electroencephalogr Clin Neurophysiol 1980;50:100.
30. Facco E, Martini A, Zuccarello M, Chiaranda M, Trincia G, Ori C, Giron GP. Auditory brainstem responses in post-traumatic comatose patients: assessment of brainstem damage and prognostic implications. Intensive Care Med 1983;9:194.
31. Klug N. Brainstem auditory evoked potentials in syndromes of decerebration, the bulbar syndrome and in central death. J Neurol 1982;227:219–28.
32. Anziska BJ, Cracco RQ. Short latency somatosensory evoked potentials in brain dead patients. Arch Neurol 1980;37:222–25.
33. de la Torre JC. Evaluation of brain death using somatosensory evoked potentials. Biol Psychiatr 1981;16:931–35.
34. Rumpl E, Prugger M, Gerstenbrand F, Hackl JM, Pallua A. Central somatosensory conduction time and short latency somatosensory evoked potentials in post-traumatic coma. Electroencephalogr Clin Neurophysiol 1983;56:583–96.
35. Anziska BJ, Cracco RQ. Short latency somatosensory evoked potentials in patients with focal neurological disease. Electroencephalogr Clin Neurophysiol 1980;49:227–39.
36. Arezzo J, Legatt AD, Vaughan HG. Topography and intracranial sources of somatosensory evoked potentials in the monkey: I. Early components. Electroencephalogr Clin Neurophysiol 1979;46:155–72.
37. Chiappa KH, Young RR, Goldie WD. Origins of the components of human short-latency somatosensory evoked responses (SER). Neurology 1979;29:598.
38. Jones SJ. Short latency potentials recorded from the neck and scalp following median nerve stimulation in man. Electroencephalogr Clin Neurophysiol 1977;43:853–63.
39. Noel P, Desmedt JE. Somatosensory cerebral evoked potentials after vascular lesions of the brain-stem and diencephalon. Brain 1975;98:113–28.
40. Kritchevsky M, Wiederholt WC. Short latency somatosensory evoked responses in man. Arch Neurol 1978;35:706–11.
41. Hume AL, Cant BR. Conduction time in central somatosensory pathways in man. Electroencephalogr Clin Neurophysiol 1978;45:361–75.
42. Cracco RQ, Cracco JB. Somatosensory evoked potential in man: far field potentials. Electroencephalogr Clin Neurophysiol 1976;41:460–66.
43. Allison T, Wood CC, McCarthy G, Hume AL, Goff WR. Short-latency somatosensory evoked potentials in man, monkey, cat and rat: comparative latency analysis. In: Courjon J, Mauguière F, Revol M, eds. Clinical applications of evoked potentials in neurology. New York: Raven Press, 1982;303–11.
44. Morillo LE, Tullock JW, Gumnit RJ, Snyder BD. Compressed spectral array patterns following cardiopulmonary arrest. A preliminary report. Arch Neurol 1983;40:287–89.
45. Karnaze DS, Marshall LF, Bickford RG. EEG monitoring of clinical coma: the compressed spectral array. Neurology (NY) 1982;32:289–92.
46. Burgess R, Cant BR, Hume AL, Priestley CL, Shaw NA. Cerebral monitoring by compressed spectral array. New Zealand Med J 1977;86:521–23.
47. Cant BR, Shaw NA. Monitoring by compressed spectral array in prolonged coma. Neurology (Cleveland) 1984;34:35–39.
48. Bricolo A, Turazzi S, Faccioli F, Dorizzi F, Sciarretta G, Erculiani P. Clinical application of compressed spectral array in long-term EEG monitoring for comatose patients. Electroencephalogr Clin Neurophysiol 1978;45:211–25.

49. Levy WJ, Shapiro HM, Maruchak G, Meathe E. Automated EEG processing for intraoperative monitoring: a comparison of techniques. Anesthesiology 1980;53:223–36.
50. Levy WJ. Intraoperative EEG patterns: Implications for EEG monitoring. Anesthesiology 1984;60:430–34.
51. Grundy BL, Lina A, Procopio PT, Janetta PJ. Reversible evoked potential changes with contraction of the VIIIth cranial nerve. Anes and Anal 1981;60:835–38.
52. Taylor MJ, Houston BD, Lowry NJ. Recovery of auditory brain-stem responses after a severe hypoxic ischemic insult. NEJM 1983;19:1169–70.

Chapter 11

Auditory Assessment of Neural Trauma

H. Gustav Mueller
Roy K. Sedge
Andres M. Salazar

Clinical and research reports have accumulated since the 1970s suggesting that audiologists and auditory tests are assuming a role of increasing importance in the assessment, management, and rehabilitation of the neural trauma patient. The audiologic evaluation of these patients is broad in scope and to a large extent can be categorized into three different areas: (1) observation of brain stem function using auditory evoked response (AER) testing, (2) assessment of the peripheral auditory system using pure-tone and speech material, and (3) evaluation of central auditory processing capabilities using difficult speech messages.

Although some overlap exists among these categories, they represent different test batteries that are administered with different questions in mind. In addition, because of the diversity of responses required from the patient, the tests are normally given at subsequent stages during the treatment and rehabilitation processes.

AER testing, most frequently including auditory brain stem response (ABR) and middle-latency responses, is sometimes the first formal auditory test administered to the head-injured patient. The popularity and sophistication of AERs has grown tremendously in recent years, and the full potential of these auditory tests has not been realized. AERs have been demonstrated to be successful, to varying degrees, in predicting the outcome of neural trauma, detecting specific injury to nerve VIII or the brain stem, evaluating overall brain stem function, determining brain death, and estimating the degree of peripheral hearing impairment [1,2]. A description of AER procedures and a discussion of their utility with the neural trauma patient were presented in Chapters 9 and 10.

The opinions and assertions contained herein are the private views of the authors and are not to be construed as official or as reflecting the views of the Department of the Army or the Department of Defense.

Assessment of the status of the peripheral auditory system is a second area of importance. Otologic injuries such as perforation of the tympanic membrane, ossicular discontinuity, oval or round window fistulae, temporal bone fracture, or nerve VIII damage occur frequently in head injury. Consequently, peripheral hearing impairment, either conductive or sensorineural, is common [1,3]. Most peripheral auditory tests, however, require a response from the patient. When the patient cannot respond, AERs can be used to estimate hearing sensitivity. This procedure does have some limitations in frequency specificity and also because abnormal AERs due to peripheral hearing loss are often difficult to distinguish from abnormal responses due to neural injury. Immittance audiometry can also be conducted with the nonresponsive patient. The components of this procedure (tympanometry, ipsilateral and contralateral acoustic reflex testing) can be used to measure middle ear function, estimate hearing sensitivity, and assess the integrity of cranial nerves VII and VIII and the caudal brain stem. If the patient is responsive, traditional methods of auditory testing can be used. These methods include the measurement of pure-tone hearing sensitivity for air conduction (via earphones) or bone conduction (via vibrator on the mastoid process) and the measurement of speech recognition—e.g., the ability to recognize monosyllabic words presented at a fixed level above auditory threshold.

The results of the peripheral auditory battery are helpful in the management of the head-injured patient throughout the treatment and rehabilitation process. First, an otologic or neuro-otologic pathology may be detected that requires immediate medical attention. Second, if a significant hearing impairment is present, necessary steps must be taken to facilitate communication with the patient. This may involve an amplification device or, in the case of a unilateral hearing loss, directing speech toward the nonimpaired ear. Finally, during the rehabilitation period, it is likely that the patient will be administered several tests in the areas of neuropsychology and speech-language pathology. Many of these tests involve speech discrimination tasks, where even a relatively mild high frequency hearing impairment can substantially alter the test outcome. Knowledge of the patient's hearing thresholds, therefore, is helpful, if not mandatory, when these tests are administered.

A final battery of audiologic tests, which is the focus of this chapter, includes those designed to assess central auditory processing. The majority of these tests requires the patient to identify a speech message that has been made difficult to understand through distortion, compression, or adding a competing noise or a competing presentation mode. Obviously, this type of testing requires an alert and responsive patient, and, therefore, cannot always be conducted. The results of the central auditory nervous system (CANS) battery, however, are useful in detecting injury to the auditory areas of the brain stem or cortex, monitoring recovery of auditory processing skills, and providing a framework for counseling the patient concerning his communication capabilities. The importance of the CANS battery in patient counseling is sometimes overlooked. During the rehabilitation period following trauma, some patients report difficulty understanding speech. Quite frequently, however, traditional audiometry reveals normal hearing sensitivity and speech recognition. CANS testing may reveal subtler auditory processing deficits and may substantiate that the complaints of the patient are warranted.

Since 1980, as part of the Vietnam Head Injury Study (VHIS) at Walter Reed Army Medical Center, we have studied more than 500 patients who sustained penetrating head injuries in Vietnam between 1967 and 1971. This chapter includes a discussion of the CANS test results for these patients with long-standing documented brain injury, including a comparison of how these findings relate to previous research using CANS testing with other types of brain injuries or diseases.

CENTRAL AUDITORY TEST BATTERY

In the mid 1950s, Italian researchers demonstrated that depressed scores for distorted speech were observed in the ear contralateral to a temporal lobe injury [4,5], and since that time, degraded speech has been the primary stimulus for CANS evaluation. In general, even when the auditory areas of the temporal lobe are involved, pure-tone or traditional speech recognition testing does not present a sufficiently difficult processing task, and consequently, the results of these tests usually are normal. CANS tests, therefore, are designed to reduce the redundancy of speech so that normals will continue to perform relatively well but individuals who also experience a reduction of redundancy of the CANS will perform poorly. Numerous tests have been devised since the 1950s for the detection of CANS injury. Eight of these CANS tests were chosen for use in the VHIS. The tests were selected to provide a range of neuroanatomic sensitivity level, stimulus type, response mode and degree of difficulty. A brief review of these CANS tests is provided. More detailed reports of auditory test protocols and review articles describing these and other CANS tests are available [6,7,8,9].

CANS tests, to some extent, can be categorized according to the neuroanatomic level of the CANS where they have been found to be the most sensitive—i.e., the brain stem or the auditory cortex. For the most part, brain stem tests measure neural synchrony or fusion, whereas cortical tests involve separation tasks. The level of difficulty of the tests also must be carefully chosen to correspond with the stage of recovery of the patient. For the VHIS, individuals were tested 12 to 14 yr following their injury, and therefore, a wide range of brain stem and cortical tests easily could be administered.

Brain Stem Tests

In addition to ABR, which is not part of this discussion, three tests designed to measure brain stem function were included in the battery: acoustic reflexes, masking level differences (MLDs), and the Synthetic Sentence Identification (SSI) test.

Acoustic Reflexes

Previously mentioned as part of the peripheral auditory battery, acoustic reflexes also provide information regarding the integrity of the auditory centers
of the caudal brain stem. Contralateral and ipsilateral acoustic reflex testing
is normally conducted at frequencies of 500 to 4000 Hz. The response observed
is a time-locked change in middle ear compliance following acoustic stimulation.
The trans-brain-stem reflex arc includes the primary afferent spiral ganglion,
nerve VIII, cochlear nuclei (primarily ventral), and the medial superior olive.
Brain stem damage can result in absent reflexes or reflexes above the normal
70 to 105 dB range. Abnormal decay of the reflex also may be present.
Additional differential information is obtained from the ipsilaterally-elicited
reflex because the arc of this response is believed to be less dependent on the
olivary complex. The acoustic reflex test has an advantage over the other tests
mentioned here in that no behavioral response from the patient is required.
Interpretation is sometimes difficult, however, if middle ear function is not
normal or if a severe peripheral hearing impairment exists.

Masking Level Differences

The masking level difference (MLD) test requires an individual to identify
speech or a pure tone in the presence of masking noise [10]. For the VHIS
protocol, binaural MLDs were conducted for 500 Hz and 1000 Hz (masking
noise presented at 80 dB sound pressure level). Separate measures were taken
for both tone and noise in phase (SoNo), tone in phase and noise 180° out of
phase (SoN$_\pi$), and tone 180° antiphasic with noise in phase (S$_\pi$No). The MLD,
expressed in decibels, is the difference between the antiphasic and the SoNo
thresholds.

   Normal subjects usually demonstrate an MLD of 7 to 16 dB for a 500
Hz tone, with mean values of 9 to 12 dB. Individuals with brain stem injury
may show substantially reduced MLDs (e.g., 4 dB or more below normal
mean), and in some extreme instances, no improvement in threshold for the
antiphasic conditions is observed—i.e., an MLD of 0 dB. The neuroanatomic
structures that are believed to be responsible for the MLD lie in the ponto-
medullary regions of the brain stem. The structure that is perhaps primarily
responsible for this phase and timing analysis is the superior olivary nucleus.

Synthetic Sentence Identification

The Synthetic Sentence Identification (SSI) test consists of ten sentences,
constructed as third-order approximations of real English sentences [11]. These
sentences are traditionally presented in combination with a contralateral or
ipsilateral competing message that consists of a single talker continuous dis-
course. For the VHIS protocol, the SSI was administered using an ipsilateral
presentation of the competing message at a 0 dB message to competition ratio
(see Figure 11.1A). The sentences and competition were presented at various
suprathreshold levels to construct a performance-intensity (P-I) function for

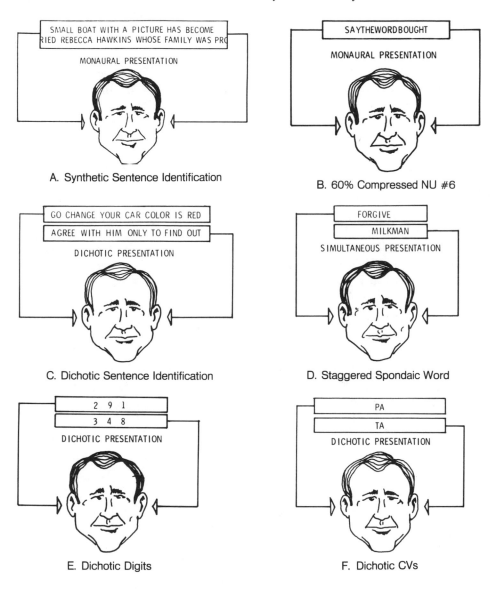

Figure 11.1 Diagrammatic representation of the presentation format of the CANS tests used in the VHIS protocol.

each patient. The sentences were presented in blocks of ten, and the patient was required to identify the number of the sentence from a printed card. Previous research using this SSI procedure has demonstrated that performance is frequently reduced in the ear ipsilateral to brain stem injury, sometimes only at the more intense presentation levels, described as rollover of the P-I function [12]. Poor performance in the ear contralateral to a temporal lobe lesion also has been described.

Cortical-Level Battery

The CANS tests discussed to this point primarily are sensitive to brain stem rather than cortical dysfunction. The majority of tests designed to assess the auditory processing capabilities of the temporal lobes or the transmission properties of the corpus callosum consists of speech material presented simultaneously to each ear. The task for the patient is usually to signal separation— i.e., to identify both speech messages. Although some monaural tests are considered to be sensitive to cortical pathology, most speech tests of higher level auditory function incorporate dichotic presentation—i.e., different speech messages presented simultaneously under earphones with careful control of timing and phase. When CANS tests are used for assessment of cortical injury, the primary crossing auditory pathway must be kept in mind. Because of this relationship, abnormal performance is expected for the ear contralateral rather than ipsilateral to temporal lobe damage. The interpretation of dichotic speech tests is based largely on the model presented by Sparks, Goodglass, and Nickel [13]. As shown in Figure 11.2, this model suggests that a dominant pathway

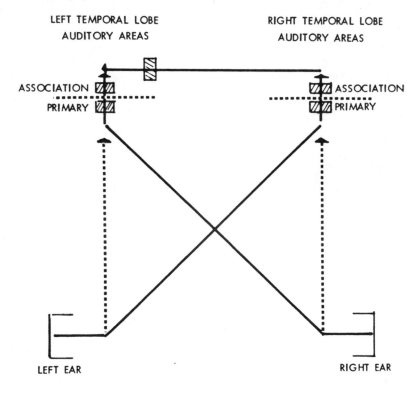

Figure 11.2 Illustration of the ipsilateral and decussating auditory pathways to the temporal lobe and across the corpus callosum. The slashed boxes represent areas where lesions may cause reduced dichotic performance (From Sparks, et al. [13]).

exists to each temporal lobe that can suppress the ipsilateral signal, that final processing occurs in the left temporal lobe, and that lesions along this pathway can reduce the performance for either the right or left ear or both. Observe that this model also would explain the reduced left ear score that has sometimes been observed when corpus callosum injury is present [14,15].

Five CANS tests were chosen for the VHIS cortical-level battery. One of these, compressed speech, is a monaural test, while the other four tests involve dichotic presentation. The dichotic tests selected provide a range of difficulty varying from the identification of sentence material to recognition of consonant-vowel nonsense syllables.

Compressed Speech

The compressed speech test utilized consists of a 60% time-compressed version of the Northwestern University Test #6 (NU #6) (Auditec of St. Louis recording) [16]. A fifty word list is administered to each ear separately at 40 dB sensation level (SL) (the speech recognition threshold, see Figure 11.1B). At this presentation level, normals usually perform in the 65 to 80% range. Previous research with monosyllabic compressed speech tests has shown that decreased performance occurs in the ear contralateral to a temporal lobe injury. This appears to be more true, however, for diffuse lesions, and individuals with discrete lesions or injury may perform normally [17].

The 60% compressed NU #6 test represents the only monaural test in the cortical-level battery. Although dichotic tests have been found to be more effective, it is useful to have at least one monaural test for patients with unilateral hearing impairment. In addition, a comparison of monaural and dichotic CANS tests may sometimes assist in differentiating corpus callosum from temporal lobe dysfunction. Although other monaural tests such as filtered speech or speech-in-noise were not used in this protocol, research suggests that these tests would provide similar information as 60% compressed speech.

Dichotic Sentence Identification

The Dichotic Sentence Identification (DSI) test is one of four dichotic tests used in this battery [18]. The DSI utilizes six of the ten sentences of the previously discussed SSI test. The sentences are paired and presented dichotically (see Figure 11.1C) as opposed to the ipsilateral-competing message condition used for the SSI. The patient is required to identify each sentence presented. Normals are expected to score relatively high (mean performance = 94%) with no significant difference between ears. The DSI was designed, at least in part, to overcome some of the influence of peripheral hearing loss on dichotic speech measures. Studies have shown that even relatively mild high frequency hearing loss can significantly reduce CANS test scores, serving to complicate test interpretation [9]. Limited research suggests that the DSI is at least somewhat resistant to high frequency hearing impairment yet maintains sensitivity for CANS dysfunction [18].

Staggered Spondaic Word

The Staggered Spondaic Word (SSW) is perhaps the most frequently used dichotic test [19]. For this procedure, the patient is presented two-syllable words (spondees), one to each ear, aligned so that the last syllable of the first word competes with the first syllable of the second word (see Figure 11.1D). The lead ear is alternated throughout the presentation of forty pairs of words. The SSW is scored by calculating correct responses for each ear, with special attention given to the competing portions. Additional scoring methods include determination of order effect—i.e., errors on the lead spondee versus the lag spondee; ear effect—i.e., errors when the right ear is the lead ear versus when the left ear is leading; and reversals—i.e., the number of times a patient answers all or part of the lag word before the lead word.

For this protocol, the SSW list EC was administered at 50 dB SL. Normals typically score above 90% for both the right and left ear competing conditions, with slightly higher scores for the right ear. Significantly reduced scores in the contralateral ear are expected when temporal lobe injury is present [20]. The most pronounced effect usually occurs when the left posterior temporal lobe is injured [21]. Some reports have indicated that ear effects and order effects correspond to the degree and location of temporal lobe involvement [20,22].

Dichotic Digits

The majority of early research on dichotic listening with normal and abnormal brains utilized dichotic digits as the test stimulus [23,24,25]. Although different in composition, the level of difficulty of the dichotic digit test is relatively equal to the competing portions of the SSW. In the traditional manner, this test consists of the numbers one through nine (excluding seven) presented dichotically in groups of three (see Figure 11.1E). The patient is required to report back the six numbers presented (three from each ear). For the VHIS protocol, twenty-four dichotic presentations (seventy-two pairings) are delivered at a level of 60 dB hearing level (HL). In recent years, Musiek and colleagues have described the use of a dichotic digit test where the digits were presented in groups of two rather than three [26]. When this procedure is used, the patient must only remember four numbers instead of six, which may be an advantage when memory deficits are present. In the present study, the dichotic digit test was administered only if the patient could demonstrate the ability to recall six digits. Normals usually score near 90%, with a 2 to 5% group advantage for the right ear. Like the SSW, abnormal performance for dichotic digits is expected in the ear contralateral to temporal lobe injury.

Dichotic Consonant-Vowel

The dichotic test that has the greatest similarity between presentation items, closely controls the timing of these items, and consequently is the most difficult is the dichotic consonant-vowel (CV) test [27]. This dichotic test consists of the voiced stop consonants /b,d,g/ and their unvoiced counterparts /p,t,k/ paired with the vowel /a/ (see Figure 11.1F). The syllables are paired and presented dichotically in a block of thirty (all possible pairings) at 60 dB HL. The patient is required to identify which two of the six CVs were presented (some clinicians/researchers have used a directed ear response mode).

Several methods are available for scoring the CVs. For the VHIS dichotic CV data described in this chapter, scores are presented in the same manner as the SSW and dichotic digits—i.e., percent correct of total items presented to each ear. One additional measure, double corrects (both right and left ear correct for a single presentation), also is discussed.

The difficulty of the dichotic CVs is reflected in the performance of normals, who usually score 60 to 80% for the right ear and 50 to 65% for the left. As indicated by these mean values, right ear scores are typically 10 to 15% better than the left ear, although considerable individual variation exists.

Based on the research of Cullen et al [28] and others, dichotic CV performance for brain-injured individuals can be summarized as follows:

1. Right temporal lobe injury results in reduced left ear performance and slightly improved right ear performance.
2. Left temporal lobe injury results in substantially reduced right ear performance and slightly reduced left ear scores.
3. Corpus callosum injury results in markedly reduced left ear scores and improved right ear performance.

As mentioned, the CANS battery presented here represents a range of difficulty believed to be appropriate for the subjects of the VHIS. In clinical practice, it may not always be feasible to deliver a battery this extensive. In these instances, the clinician must select specific tests that are appropriate for the suspected level of CANS dysfunction, easy enough for the patient to perform, and difficult enough to retain sensitivity.

VIETNAM HEAD INJURY STUDY GROUP RESULTS

This section presents some of the preliminary analyses for CANS tests for the VHIS subjects. Many of the group summaries were conducted at different stages of data collection, and therefore, the number of subjects in each group varies slightly among the CANS tests described. For most of the tests, the results of the head-injured subjects are compared to those of a control group. The control group consists of veterans who served in Vietnam but did not sustain head injury. This group is matched for age, amount and type of service in Vietnam, and scores on cognitive testing obtained on entry into the military.

Several subjects in both the control and head-injured groups have peripheral hearing impairment. For some cases, the impairment is quite severe and appears secondary to the injury. For most cases, however, the hearing loss is limited to the high frequencies and can be attributed to prolonged noise exposure from military weapon fire. To account for the possible effects of hearing impairment on CANS test outcome, the data presented in this section only include the results for subjects scoring 94% or higher for conventional monosyllabic word recognition testing (NU #6). Previous analysis of these data has shown that hearing impairment had the most substantial effect on the dichotic CVs and the compressed speech test.

Brain Stem Battery

As might be expected from this patient population, the CANS tests designed to detect brain stem dysfunction were relatively normal when group results were analyzed. Although it is usually assumed that temporal lobe damage will have little effect on lower level auditory processing, surprisingly little research has been conducted in this area.

Research by Gelfand and Silman has shown acoustic reflex thresholds remain normal when cortical injury is present [29]. In general, the VHIS group data agree with these findings. Although specific individual analysis may reveal significant interactions, group findings can be summarized as follows:

1. Reflex thresholds for the head-injured group are similar to that of published normative data.
2. Reflex thresholds for the head-injured group are similar to those for the control group.
3. Reflex thresholds are similar among individuals with different injury sites (e.g., parietal lobe versus temporal lobe).

Like the acoustic reflex, research studying MLDs for brain-injured subjects is also limited. The results of at least two different reports, however, have suggested that higher level brain stem or cortical dysfunction has little or no effect on the phase and timing processing necessary for the MLD test [30,31]. The results of MLD testing with the VHIS population support this notion. Table 11.1 presents the mean binaural MLDs for 500 Hz for forty-three

Table 11.1 Means and Standard Deviations for 500 Hz MLD

	Controls	Left Posterior Temporal Lobe Injury	Right Posterior Temporal Lobe Injury
Number	50	43	40
Mean	9.9 dB	9.2 dB	9.1 dB
S.D.	2.3 dB	2.3 dB	2 dB

individuals with right posterior temporal lobe injury and forty individuals with left posterior temporal lobe injury. As can be observed, the mean values are only slightly below that of the control group, and do not vary significantly among groups ($p > .05$). A limited number of individuals with high frequency hearing impairment are present in each group (including the controls), which may account for the fact that all mean values occurred 1 to 2 dB below previously reported normative data [32].

The third CANS test included in the brain stem battery was the SSI with ipsilateral competing message (ICM). As with acoustic reflexes and MLDs, SSI-ICM results for the VHIS subjects typically have been normal. In administering this test to eighty consecutive subjects, rollover for the P-I function was only observed in two cases, and only one case demonstrated overall depressed scores. A review of the CT scans of these three cases suggested that the abnormal performance could be attributed to damage to the contralateral temporal lobe rather than brain stem damage on the ipsilateral side. Although the SSI-ICM is reportedly sensitive to temporal lobe injury [7] and therefore could be considered as part of the cortical test battery, the sentence identification task with ipsilateral competition does not appear to be difficult enough for the majority of subjects studied in this research project.

In summary, normal findings were obtained for the CANS tests geared toward the evaluation of the auditory centers of the brain stem. Given the recovery stage of the VHIS subjects, these findings are not surprising, and these psychophysical data are in good agreement with the ABR results for the same subjects. These findings, however, are nevertheless interesting because they lend support to previous research regarding the relationship of cortical injury on acoustic reflex and MLD results.

Cortical-Level Battery

The cortical-level battery has been the primary emphasis of test administration and interpretation for the VHIS auditory protocol. An issue of particular interest has been the influence of injury at specific neuroanatomical areas on CANS test performance. The group results presented here are discussed relative to this relationship.

Compressed Speech

As mentioned, compressed speech is the only monaural CANS test included in the VHIS battery. Since many of the VHIS subjects have moderate to severe unilateral hearing impairments, this test sometimes has been the only means of obtaining information regarding auditory processing skills, albeit only from one ear.

Compressed speech scores from both ears were compared to various injury sites (e.g., temporal lobe, parietal lobe, etc.) for both hemispheres. The only injury area groups demonstrating scores significantly below those of the controls were the individuals with right and left posterior temporal lobe injury. As can be observed from Table 11.2, even the mean performance for these cases is not substantially lower than the control group. A trend toward a contralateral ear effect appears present, but again, only small differences exist between ears. Also displayed in Table 11.2 are the difference scores—i.e., the difference between the 60% compressed NU #6 score and the subject's non-compressed NU #6 score. As with the mean data, aside from the greater variability associated with the contralateral ear, these different score results do not vary substantially from the control group data. In general, it appears that 60% compressed speech does not present a difficult enough processing task for the majority of the VHIS subjects, and performance, therefore, remains in the normal range. The discrete nature of most of the injuries and the multiple processing pathways available to a monaural speech message probably are responsible for this finding.

Dichotic Sentence Identification

The DSI uses sentence material and for this reason is perhaps the easiest of the dichotic tests used in this protocol. Because the DSI was only developed in 1983 [18], it has received limited use with the VHIS subjects. In an attempt to compare the sensitivity of the DSI to other dichotic tests, the DSI was administered as part of the auditory protocol to thirty consecutive subjects of the VHIS. Because many of these subjects had injury outside the auditory processing areas, normal performance was obtained for all dichotic tests.

Table 11.3 illustrates the findings for thirteen subjects who scored abnormally on at least one test (there was no case where abnormal performance only was present for the DSI). As can be observed in Table 11.3, DSI scores appear to be related to the frequency with which performance on other tests is abnormal. For example, the three cases that show abnormal scores for all three of the other dichotic tests also have abnormal performance for the DSI. DSI scores, however, are normal for the remaining ten cases. This finding suggests, at least for our limited sample, that the sensitivity of the DSI is lower than some other dichotic tests used in this protocol. Recall, however, that the DSI was not necessarily designed as a highly sensitive dichotic test but as a CANS test that can be used when peripheral hearing loss is present. Current analysis of the VHIS data is directed toward this topic.

Staggered Spondaic Word

When the VHIS subjects were grouped according to injury site, SSW scores were reduced significantly only when injury was in the left or right posterior temporal lobe. These findings were similar for dichotic digits and the dichotic CVs, and the results for all three tests are illustrated in Table 11.4. Observe that the controls' variation for the SSW is much smaller than for the other two tests. This finding adds more significance to the relatively high group scores

Table 11.2 Means, Difference Scores, and Standard Deviations (percent) for 60% NU #6 Compressed Speech Results

	Controls		Left Posterior Temporal Lobe Injury		Right Posterior Temporal Lobe Injury	
	Right	*Left*	*Right*	*Left*	*Right*	*Left*
Number	40	39	21	20	26	27
Mean	85.5	83.6	76.1	81.5	79.2	76.9
S.D.	6.4	9.7	21.1	8.8	10.3	14.3
Difference score	14.3	15.5	21.1	16.9	17.5	19.6
S.D.	6.2	9.1	20.5	9.1	9.7	13.4

Note: Difference score is 60% compressed NU #6 score subtracted from noncompressed NU #6 score.

Table 11.3 Dichotic Sentence Identification (DSI) Test Results for Thirteen Cases Demonstrating Abnormal Performance on Other Dichotic Tests

DSI		SSW		Dichotic Digits		Dichotic CVs	
Right	*Left*	*Right*	*Left*	*Right*	*Left*	*Right*	*Left*
100	40	X	X		X		X
87	83					X	X
93	80		X				
93	97					X	
97	97	X	X				
97	100		X				
100	100						
100	97		X			X	X
100	97						
50	60	X	X	X	X	X	
100	100		X				X
90	63	X	X	X	X	X	
93	90		X				
93	97					X	X

Note: Abnormal performance (below ninetieth percentile cutoff) designated by X.

Table 11.4 Group Means and Standard Deviations for the SSW, Dichotic Digits, and Dichotic CVs for Controls and Individuals with Left and Right Posterior Temporal Lobe Injury

Test	Controls		Left Posterior Temporal Lobe Injury		Right Posterior Temporal Lobe Injury	
	Right	*Left*	*Right*	*Left*	*Right*	*Left*
SSW						
Mean	98.7	95.2	87.6	89.3	95.6	85.2
S.D.	2.8	6.1	22.7	12.2	6.7	15.4
Dichotic digits						
Mean	91	88.5	80.4	74.8	90	82.6
S.D.	15.2	15.8	18.9	26.9	8.2	14.6
Dichotic CVs						
Mean	75.5	54.4	50.8	54.2	79.3	34.1
S.D.	14.6	18	28.9	36.6	21.3	22.6

Note: Mean scores represent percent correct for each dichotic test for the right and left ears.

that were obtained when injury was present. The left hemisphere–right hemisphere relationship expected from the dichotic model appears to be present; that is, left hemisphere injury caused poorer performance for both ears, with the greatest effect for the right ear. Right temporal lobe injury, in contrast, resulted in poorer performance for the left ear, but the right ear scores were essentially normal.

A second area of interest concerning the SSW results was the analysis of the types of errors (the ear effects and order effects discussed earlier). While some authors have suggested that this type of analysis differentiates injury sites [20,22], other reports have questioned the validity of this approach [33,34,35].

The analysis for ear effect for the right and left posterior temporal lobe injuries is displayed in Table 11.5. The mean values are based on percent correct, and the significant effects are determined by the number of errors for a presentation format—i.e., right ear first (REF) or left ear first (LEF). A difference in error rate of five or more is considered significant. Observe that group performance is relatively equal for the REF and LEF presentation formats. When the individual distributions of ear effects are compared, it appears that ear effects are more frequent when injury is in the left rather than the right hemisphere; however, no clear REF versus LEF relationship is present. The work of Katz suggests that individuals with posterior temporal lobe injury should demonstrate more errors for the REF condition [20]. As seen in Table 11.5, these data fail to support this relationship.

The analysis for order effect is shown in Table 11.6. As with ear effect, the majority of subjects did not demonstrate a significant effect, and the greatest number of significant effects (error difference of five or more between the first and second spondee) was noted for the left hemisphere. Unlike the ear effect results, however, there appears to be a clear pattern of the order effect analysis. As seen from Table 11.6, when a significant effect occurs, the greatest number of errors is usually present for the first spondee. This finding is especially interesting since it is in direct opposition to the pattern that other authors have stated should be present for posterior temporal lobe injury [20,22]. Obviously, more research on the SSW ear effect and order effect error analysis is necessary, and until a more definitive relationship can be established, a cautious application seems warranted.

Dichotic Digits

The dichotic digit results for the left and right temporal lobe injury groups are shown in Table 11.4. In general, the group performance is similar to the pattern demonstrated for the SSW. Somewhat at variance, however, are the findings for the left hemisphere injury group, showing the greatest reduction in performance for the left (ipsilateral) ear rather than for the right (contralateral) ear. The dichotic digits test results also revealed an interesting pattern when compared with the SSW and the dichotic CVs relative to injury site. Table 11.7 shows the distribution of significant associations between injury area and SSW,

Table 11.5 Mean Performance for SSW Right Ear First (REF) and Left Ear First (LEF) Presentation Formats and Distribution of Significant Ear Effects

Injury Site	Number	Mean Percent Correct		Distribution of Ear Effect			
		REF	*LEF*	*No Effect*	*REF > LEF*	*LEF > REF*	
Right posterior temporal Right area of Heschl's gyrus	37	94.7	92.6	30	1	6	
	18	92.8	89.2	13	1	4	
Left posterior temporal Left area of Heschl's gyrus	39	91.5	92	21	8	10	
	22	89.1	90.7	11	6	5	

Note: Difference of five or more errors between REF and LEF conditions.

Table 11.6 Mean Performance for SSW Order Effects for First Spondee and Second Spondee and Distribution of Significant Order Effects

Injury Site	Number	Mean Percent Correct		Distribution of Order Effect		
		First Spondee	Second Spondee	No Effect	First > Second	Second > First
Right posterior temporal	37	92.5	94.7	29	7	1
Right area of Heschl's gyrus	18	89.7	92.3	12	5	1
Left posterior temporal	39	89.7	93.8	24	13	2
Left area of Heschl's gyrus	22	87.4	92.4	12	9	1

Note: Difference of five or more errors between first and second spondee presented.

Table 11.7 Significant Associations ($p < .01$) between Right Ear and Left Ear Dichotic Test Score and Injury Site

Injury Site	Dichotic CVs		SSW		Dichotic Digits	
	Right	*Left*	*Right*	*Left*	*Right*	*Left*
Right injury						
Temporal		X				
Anterior		X				
Posterior		X				
Parietal					X	
Frontal						
Occipital						
Left injury						
Temporal	X		X	X	X	X
Anterior			X		X	
Posterior	X		X		X	
Parietal			X		X	
Frontal						
Occipital					X	

Note: Significant associations are designated by X.

digit, and CV dichotic scores for the right and left ears. Analysis was conducted using a two-tailed Fisher exact test of independence in a two-by-two table. Associations, which are marked by X on the chart, are significant at the .01 level.

The findings for the dichotic CVs are rather straightforward. Observe that the significant relationships only are present between temporal lobe injury and the contralateral ear dichotic score. No significant relationship was observed between right or left CV score and injury to other brain areas. As opposed to the CV results, the findings for the SSW and dichotic digits are not as easily explained. First, neither the SSW nor digit scores were associated significantly with right temporal lobe injury. In fact, the only significant finding for right injury was the right digit score paired with the parietal lobe, an ipsilateral rather than contralateral effect. For left injury, the expected association for the right ear score and temporal lobe injury was obtained for both tests. The right ear scores, however, also were significant for parietal lobe injury, and curiously, the right digit score was associated significantly with damage to the occipital lobe. It is possible that the memory and mnemonic processing ability required for the dichotic digits influenced these unexpected associations. It must also be kept in mind that many of these subjects have injuries to multiple lobes or multiple areas of a single lobe.

Dichotic Consonant-Vowels

The final CANS test discussed in this section is the dichotic CVs. Although some consider this test too difficult to be included in a CANS battery, more than 90% of the VHIS subjects were able to understand the test and respond appropriately. The group results for the CVs are shown in Table 11.4 and correspond to the expected findings based on the dichotic model and previous research in this area. Of interest is the mean right ear score for individuals with right posterior temporal lobe damage, which shows group performance to be better than that of the controls. This improved right ear effect is demonstrated more clearly for CVs than for the other dichotic tests, probably because of the more precise control of timing for the CV material.

In addition to the right and left ear percent correct scores, a second area of interest includes the number of double correct responses (correct report of both CVs for a dichotic presentation). Table 11.8 shows the distribution of percent of CV double corrects for four groups: controls, head injury other than temporal lobe, left temporal lobe injury, and right temporal lobe injury. Observe that when the injury is not in the temporal lobe, the distribution of double correct responses follows a pattern very similar to that of the control groups. When injury is in the temporal lobe, however, the pattern changes considerably, and the majority of individuals in these groups has less than 10% double correct responses. Although one might expect that left hemisphere damage would affect double correct responses more than injury to the right, this effect is not present for this sample. These findings are encouraging and

Table 11.8 Percent Distribution of Double Correct CV Responses for Controls, Head Injured Excluding Temporal Lobe, and Left and Right Temporal Lobe Injury Groups

Group	Number	Percent of CV Double Correct Responses					
		0–10%	*10–20%*	*20–30%*	*30–40%*	*40–50%*	*> 50%*
Controls	58	10	16	17	28	16	14
Head Injured excluding temporal lobe injury	115	16	22	26	14	15	8
Left temporal lobe injury	34	39	33	17	9	3	0
Right temporal lobe injury	36	35	30	18	9	3	6

suggest that double correct responses may be helpful in assessing the overall auditory processing capabilities of an individual.

This brief report of group findings for the VHIS subjects has shown that for most tests, performance has paralleled the outcome expected from previous research in this area. The availability of detailed CT scan analysis has allowed for relatively precise definition of injury areas and the study of the relationship of this injury to test performance. Further study of injury to discrete temporal lobe areas may reveal even more direct relationships to auditory processing.

CASES

All subjects participating in the VHIS were administered CT scans. The scans were performed on a General Electric 8800 scanner, at a 25° angle to Reid's baseline at 5 mm intervals, yielding approximately 22 to 24 slices per subject. The following cases are presented to demonstrate the relationship between brain injury based on CT scan analysis and behavioral performance on CANS tests.

Case 1

A 35-yr-old white man sustained a penetrating craniocerebral wound in 1968. The point of entry was in the right temporal region. Initial surgical treatment consisted of a right temporal craniectomy with wound debridement and resection of a small portion of the right temporal lobe. He had no complications postoperatively. CT scan (Figure 11.3) revealed a right temporal craniectomy with an underlying right temporal lobe defect, extending toward the temporal pole but sparing the most anterior portion. Minimal extension of the lesion is seen along the inferior temporal gyrus. The most anterior frontal opercular cortex is also involved. The

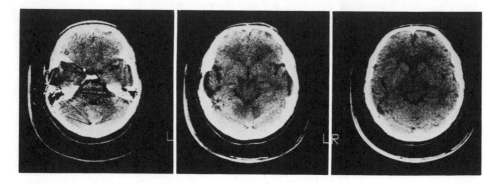

Figure 11.3   CT scan analysis for Case 1. Projections (left to right) are 25 mm, 35 mm, and 45 mm from reference.

insula, basal ganglia, and occipital lobe are spared. Speech and language evaluation was normal, although some dysgraphia and dysnomia were noted. Visual-spatial perception capacity and memory were mildly impaired.

Peripheral auditory testing revealed normal hearing sensitivity and excellent speech recognition scores bilaterally. Acoustic reflexes were present for all stimulus conditions at 80 to 95 dB (500 to 2000 Hz). The 500 Hz MLD was 9 dB. Dichotic test results are presented in Table 11.9. Observe that for all three tests, performance was equal to that of the controls. The findings for this case, which are consistent with those for other VHIS cases with similar injury, reveal that when injury is limited to the anterior portions of the temporal lobe, performance for all auditory tests including dichotic processing tasks is frequently normal. This appears to be especially true when involvement is discrete and in the right hemisphere.

Case 2

Case 2 is a 35-yr-old white man who sustained two penetrating fragment wounds to the left frontal area in 1969. Skull X-ray revealed multiple fragment wounds in both hemispheres and in-driven bone. His initial surgery included a left frontal craniectomy with debridement of necrotic brain tissue and removal of bone and metallic fragments. Postoperatively, he was lethargic, mildly aphasic, and had a right hemiparesis. Ten days postoperatively, he was found to have a purulent meningitis. The wound was reopened and a small dural leak was noted anteriorly and repaired. He recovered uneventfully. Aside from a significant dysnomia, the speech and language testing was within normal limits. The patient's area of major cognitive impairment is in verbal memory. CT scan revealed a left frontal cranioplasty and an underlying full thickness defect (Figure 11.4). A left frontal convexity defect is seen with involvement of white matter beneath the atrophic mesial cortex. Ex vacuo enlargement of the ventricular system is seen, and the anterior ventricular structures are shifted toward the defect. Multiple metallic fragments can be observed both within this defect and extending across the midline

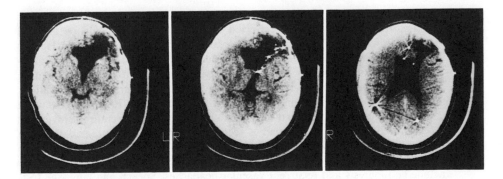

Figure 11.4   CT scan analysis for Case 2. Projections (left to right) are 40 mm, 50 mm, and 65 mm from reference.

into the right frontal and temporal lobes in one projection and across the ventricular system to the right parietal and parieto-occipital lobes in a separate projection. Another metallic fragment is seen near the dependent portion of the left lateral ventricular atrium. There is an area of decreased density in the corpus callosum centrally. Anteriorly there is also an area of apparent calcification surrounding one of the metallic fragments in the rostrum.

Hearing sensitivity for Case 2 was normal except for a mild to moderate high frequency loss (above 3000 Hz) in the right ear. Speech recognition was 100% bilaterally. Acoustic reflexes were present for all test frequencies at 80 to 100 dB, and the 500 Hz MLD was 18 dB. The results for the dichotic CANS tests are shown in Table 11.9. It can be seen that for each dichotic test, left ear performance is reduced, although not always falling below the ninetieth percentile cutoff scores. Also noticeable, and perhaps more significant, are the excellent scores obtained on the dichotic tests for the right ear. This is particularly evident for the dichotic CVs, where right ear performance far exceeds that of controls. As indicated by the double correct score, all left ear correct responses were obtained in combination with a right ear correct response.

These subtle, but significant, results for Case 2 could be attributed to the right temporal lobe involvement that appears to be superior/posterior to the area of Heschl's gyrus. It is also possible that corpus callosum damage, which is suspected in this case, is preventing adequate representation of the left ear material (transferring from the right hemisphere) in the left hemisphere. This also could explain the more pronounced findings for the CV material, where timing is the most closely aligned. In some instances, monaural CANS tests are helpful in clarifying the cause of a reduced left ear dichotic speech score (i.e., if the cause is corpus callosum damage, the monaural test frequently will be normal due to the absence of competition and the intact ipsilateral pathway to the left hemisphere.) For this case, however, 60% compressed speech scores were essentially normal (right ear, 84%; left ear, 76%) but slightly more depressed for the left ear and therefore provide little assistance in interpretation.

Case 3

A 33-yr-old white man in 1969 suffered a high velocity gunshot wound to the left frontal-parietal region. He was reported to be stuporous but could be aroused and followed commands on initial examination several hours after injury. He was aphasic with a right hemiparesis at that time. He underwent an extensive craniectomy and debridement on the day of injury and underwent a second operation for removal of retained bone fragments 2 day later. Postoperative complications included delayed wound healing and meningitis. In March 1970 he underwent an acrylic cranioplasty, but this had to be removed because of infection in November 1970. The following June he had a second acrylic cranioplasty, and this one remained in place for 9 yr until 1980 when it, too, had to be removed because of a secondary infection. The patient currently has no cranioplasty. Other residuals include hemiparesis and recurrent vascular headaches. Speech and language testing revealed a moderate to severe residual mixed aphasia with deficits in all linguistic areas. There was significant reduction in verbal expression, phrase

Table 11.9 Dichotic Test Results for Cases 1 to 4, Showing Right and Left Ear Percent Correct Score and Double Correct Scores for the Dichotic CV Test

	SSW		*Dichotic Digits*		*Dichotic CVs*		*Double Correct*
Case	*Right*	*Left*	*Right*	*Left*	*Right*	*Left*	
Case 1	95	95	94	90	70	67	40
Case 2	98	82	100	86	97	27	27
Case 3	2	78	10	69	7	73	0
Case 4	65	62	72	56	33	23	0
Control group							
Mean	99	95	91	89	76	54	36
S.D.	3	6	15	16	15	18	18
Ninetieth percentile cutoff	93	89	84	73	60	31	10

Note: Control group data shown for comparison.

length, syntax, fluency, and recall. He has alexia, severe dysnomia, and oral and verbal dyspraxia. He was depressed with poor self-care and a relatively poor self-image.

CT scan (Figure 11.5) revealed an extensive left frontal-parietal lobe bone defect. The entire left frontal lobe with the exception of some damaged mesial cortex is absent as is a major portion of the left basal nuclear structures. The left temporal lobe is likewise lost anteriorly with significant defect extending posteriorly. Large portions of the parietal lobe are gone with some minimal residual parasagittal parietal cortex. Atrophic changes are seen in the left occipital lobe, which is relatively spared. Ex vacuo shift of midline structures from right to left is present, and the third ventricle is enlarged as a result of basal nuclear loss on the left. The left cerebral peduncle is markedly atrophic. The right cerebral cortex appears well maintained, with diffuse cerebellar atrophic change seen to a moderate degree.

The peripheral auditory battery for this case showed normal hearing sensitivity bilaterally through 4000 Hz, with a mild impairment at 6000 and 8000 Hz. Speech recognition was good for the left ear (96%) and slightly reduced for the right (86%). Acoustic reflexes were present at normal levels. The patient was not able to perform the MLD procedure. The results of the CANS dichotic tests are shown in Table 11.9. As can be observed, performance is extremely poor for the right ear on all three tests. This would be expected, assuming that for this patient essentially all auditory processing is occurring in the right hemisphere. Of interest is the fact that right ear performance is as good for the more difficult CV material as it is for the meaningful words of the SSW or the dichotic digits. Again, this may be due to greater control of the stimulus onset time, providing a consistent advantage for the left ear CV in the right hemisphere. This point is illustrated further by the absence of any double correct responses for the CVs. When a 90 msec right ear lead was introduced for the CV material, the left ear score was reduced to 43%, and again, no double correct scores were present. With a 90 msec left ear lead, however, performance for the left ear was 63%, and 7% double corrects were obtained.

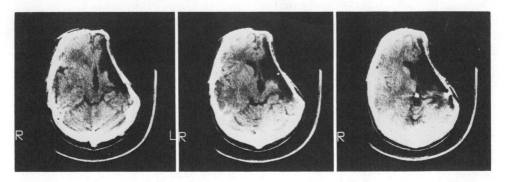

Figure 11.5   CT scan analysis for Case 3. Projections (left to right) are 40 mm, 45 mm, and 55 mm from reference.

Case 4

A 33-yr-old white man had a negative past medical history until 1967 when he suffered a mortar fragment wound to the left parietal area. He has no recollection of the injury and had a retrograde amnesia of over 1 wk, although he reportedly had no immediate loss of consciousness. The patient was described as stuporous but responding to pain and exhibited a right hemiparesis on initial examination several hours after injury. He underwent a left parietal craniectomy with debridement on the day of injury, but debridement was stopped when choroid plexus was encountered. A 5 mm metallic fragment was noted to have crossed the midline to the right parietal lobe. In a subsequent operation a retained bone fragment was removed from its position medial to the left ventricle. The second postoperative course was uneventful except for a nominal aphasia that gradually improved. Formal speech and language testing revealed a probable residual Wernicke's aphasia. There was some oral dyspraxia with oral and written dysnomia, oral and comprehension dyslexia, and moderately severe spelling deficit. Neuropsychological testing revealed an average IQ. Reasoning and problem-solving skills were impaired but the simpler nonverbal problem-solving skills were intact. Memory tests revealed a moderately severe impairment of long-term verbal memory, but nonverbal memory was relatively normal.

CT scan (Figure 11.6) revealed a left temporal occipital cranioplasty. There is a full thickness cortical deficit in the underlying left lateral temporal occipital region. There is a small missile track with multiple tiny fragments extending through the lateral ventricle atria and anterior calcarine cortex region to a large metallic fragment resting against the internal table of the skull in the right temporal occipital region. The track spares the basal ganglia structures with a possible exception of the tail of the caudate nucleus. The posterior fossa appears normal.

This patient has normal hearing through 3000 Hz bilaterally, with a mild to moderate impairment for both ears in the 4000 to 8000 Hz region. Speech recognition is excellent for both ears. Acoustic reflexes are present in the normal range for frequencies of 500 to 2000 Hz. Dichotic speech testing revealed reduced

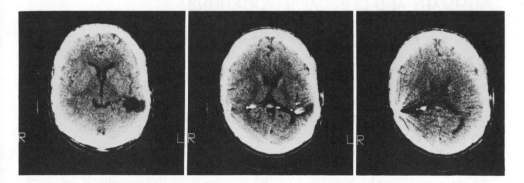

Figure 11.6 CT scan analysis for Case 4. Projections (left to right) are 50 mm, 65 mm, and 70 mm from reference.

scores for both ears for all three tests (see Table 11.9). In contrast to Cases 2 and 3, when the results for Case 4 are compared to the control data, the degree of reduction appears to be equal for both ears and for each dichotic test. The reduced performance for the right ear for this patient can be attributed with a fair degree of certainty to the left temporal lobe injury, which appears to encompass the area of Heschl's gyrus.

Speculation on the cause of the reduced performance for the left ear is more interesting, however, because at least three different explanations are tenable. First, left temporal lobe damage is known sometimes to cause an ipsilateral as well as contralateral ear effect due to the overall importance of this hemisphere in processing speech. A second possible cause, as discussed in Case 2, is corpus callosum involvement, which also can cause depressed dichotic scores for the left ear. The CT scans suggest that the metal fragments crossed near the medial area of the corpus callosum where auditory fibers are believed to pass. Finally, as evidenced by the remaining metallic fragments (see Figure 11.6), damage to the right temporal lobe also is present. Although the damaged region appears to be slightly posterior/superior to the area of Heschl's gyrus, it is possible that this injury area could be significantly affecting this patient's dichotic processing ability. Support for the latter explanation is found in the compressed speech scores, which are 16% for the right ear and 28% for the left. This severe bilateral reduction is not normally observed for either left temporal lobe or corpus callosum injury.

These illustrative cases have been presented to demonstrated some of the expected relationships between CANS tests and neuroanatomic injury site. The reader must keep in mind, however, that this testing was performed 12 to 14 yr following injury and that the patients were relatively young at the time of neural trauma. Testing conducted on more recent trauma victims may show somewhat different results, although the same test patterns, neuroanatomic relationships, and interpretation strategies would be applicable.

SUMMARY AND CLINICAL IMPLICATIONS

The group results and illustrative cases have demonstrated what information can be obtained when CANS testing is conducted with the neural trauma patient. As illustrated, the effects of brain injury on auditory processing functions can be easily measured, and significant relationships have been identified between injury site and CANS test performance. The presentation of this information is not complete, however, without a plea for cautious clinical application.

Numerous research reports have addressed the issue of sensitivity and specificity for audiologic tests [36,37,38]. These reports have primarily focused on the operating characteristics of the tests used in the peripheral auditory battery—i.e., differentiation of cochlear versus nerve VIII pathology. The same concerns of sensitivity and specificity also apply to the tests of the CANS battery.

The sensitivity of a test, on the one hand, refers to the likelihood that the test will be positive when injury is present. Specificity, on the other hand, refers to the likelihood that the test result will be normal when injury is not present. These two operating characteristics are inversely related; that is, a gain in sensitivity usually results in a loss in specificity. An ideal test would have a sensitivity and specificity of 100%. Tests that typically are used to predict the presence of a nerve VIII pathology (e.g., ABR and acoustic reflex studies) usually have been found to have a sensitivity and specificity in the 80 to 90% range.

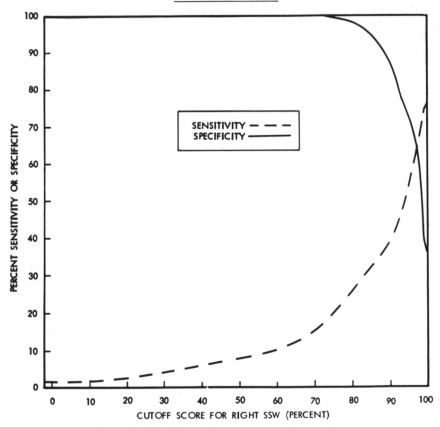

Figure 11.7   Plots of sensitivity and specificity for three dichotic tests as a function of cutoff score. Comparison is for right ear score/left posterior temporal lobe injury. A: Right SSW score. B: Right dichotic digit score. C: Right dichotic CV score.

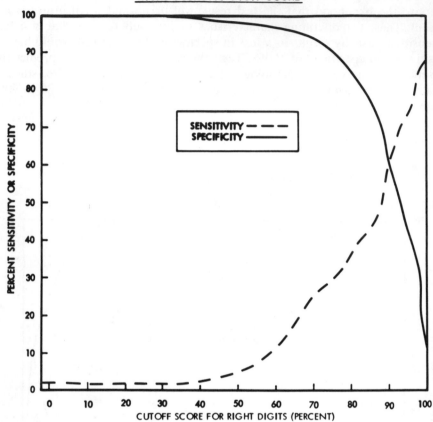

POSTERIOR TEMPORAL LOBE DAMAGED ON THE LEFT SIDE
RIGHT DICHOTIC DIGIT SCORE

Figure 11.7 (cont.)

The VHIS population provided an excellent opportunity to study the operating characteristics of CANS tests. The ear versus hemisphere relationships of auditory processing present a special challenge that does not exist when the peripheral auditory tests are studied. Figures 11.7A to C present the sensitivity and specificity results for three CANS tests for one of these relationships: the right ear score when left posterior temporal lobe damage is present. In determining sensitivity and specificity, a test score must be considered as either normal or abnormal, and therefore, the value selected as the cutoff score for normal is critical. For this reason, Figures 11.7A to C show the data ($n = 183$) plotted for all cutoff scores. The relationship between sensitivity, specificity, and cutoff score is clearly visualized.

When the functions of the three tests are compared, the relative difficulty of each test is apparent. Observe, e.g., that for the SSW, which is the easiest of the three tests, sensitivity would only reach 100% if a right ear SSW score

POSTERIOR TEMPORAL LOBE DAMAGED ON THE LEFT SIDE

RIGHT DICHOTIC CV SCORE

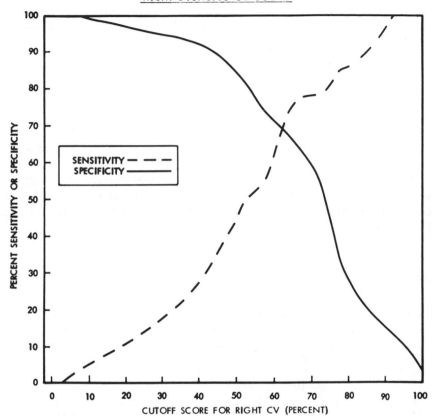

Figure 11.7 (cont.)

of 100% would be considered abnormal. By comparison, 100% sensitivity for the CVs could be obtained using a cutoff score of 92%. Unfortunately, however, this cutoff score would result in the dichotic CV test specificity's falling below 20%. If one is interested in obtaining the best possible specificity and sensitivity, then the cutoff score corresponding to the crossing point of the two functions would be selected. A review of the data presented for these three dichotic tests reveals that it is not possible to obtain high sensitivity and specificity using a single cutoff score. The best combined effectiveness appears to be present for the CV score when a 63% cutoff score is used. These findings, of course, are unique to the VHIS population studied. It is probable that higher sensitivity would result if more recent and diffuse temporal lobe injuries were studied.

These sensitivity and specificity findings point out the precautions that must be taken if these CANS tests are used to predict the presence or absence of injury rather than to describe group performance. As the role of the audiologist in the assessment of neural trauma continues to expand, it is likely that old tests will be revised and new tests will be developed. The operating characteristics for each test, however, continually must be considered whenever CANS testing is conducted.

ACKNOWLEDGMENTS

The Vietnam Head Injury study is under the auspices of the Veterans Administration [VA Contract V101 (91) M-79-31-2] with the cooperation and support of the United States Army, Navy, and Air Force.

Assistance in preparation of this manuscript was provided by Stephen C. Vance. Data collection was provided by William Beck, Brian Hill, and Sharon Fineberg. Assistance with data reduction and statistical analysis was provided by Duke Owen and Sarah Schlesselman.

REFERENCES

1. Keith RW, Jabre AF, Heerse KL. Auditory brainstem response testing in the surgical intensive care unit. Sem Hearing 1983;4:385–90.
2. Hall JW, Mackey-Hargadine J. Auditory evoked responses in severe head injury. Sem Hearing 1984;5:313–36.
3. Hall JW, Huangfu M, Gennarelli TA. Auditory function in acute severe head injury. Laryngoscope 1982;92:883–90.
4. Bocca E, Calearo C, Cassinari V. A new method for testing hearing in temporal lobe tumors: preliminary report. Acta Otolaryngol (Stockholm) 1954;44:219–21.
5. Bocca E, Calearo C, Cassinari V, Migliavacca F. Testing "cortical" hearing in temporal lobe tumors. Acta Otolaryngol (Stockholm) 1955;45:289–304.
6. Rintelmann WF, Lynn GE. Speech Stimuli for Assessment of Central Auditory Disorders. In Konkle DF, Rintelman WF, eds. Principles of Speech Audiometry Baltimore: University Park Press 1983;231–83.
7. Hall JW. Diagnostic applications of speech audiometry. Sem Hearing 1983;4:179–203.
8. Musiek FE. The evaluation of brainstem disorders using ABR and central auditory tests. Monographs in Contemporary Audiology 1983;4:1–24.
9. Mueller HG. Evaluation of central auditory function; Monosyllabic procedures. In: Katz J, ed. Handbook of clinical audiology, 3rd ed. Baltimore: Williams and Wilkins, 1985;355–82.
10. Hirsh IJ. The influence of interaural phase on interaural summation and inhibition. J Acoust Soc 1948;20:536–44.
11. Speaks CE, Jerger JF. Methods for measurement of speech identification. J Speech Hearing Res 1965;8:185–94.
12. Jerger S, Jerger JF. Auditory disorders: a manual for clinical evaluation. Boston: Little, Brown & Co., 1981.

13. Sparks R, Goodglass H, Nickel B. Ipsilateral versus contralateral extinction in dichotic listening results from hemisphere lesions. Cortex 1970;6:249–60.

14. Sparks R, Geschwind N. Dichotic listening in man after section of neocortical commissures. Cortex 1968;4:3–16.

15. Musiek FE, Kibbe K, Baran J. Neuroaudiological results from split-brain patients. Sem Hearing 1984;5:219–29.

16. Beasley D, Schwimmer S, Rintelmann WF. Intelligibility of time-compressed CNC monosyllables. J Speech Hearing Res 1972;15:340–50.

17. Kurdziel S, Noffsinger PD, Olsen W. Performance by cortical lesion patients on 40 and 60% time-compressed materials. J Audiol Soc 1976;2:3–7.

18. Fifer RJ, Jerger JF, Berlin C, Tobey EA, Campbell JC. Development of a dichotic sentence identification test for hearing impaired adults. Ear and Hearing 1983;4:300–05.

19. Katz J. The use of staggered spondaic words for assessing the integrity of the central auditory nervous system. J Auditory Res 1962;2:327–37.

20. Arnst D. Overview of the staggered spondaic word test and the competing environmental sounds test. In: Katz J, Arnst D, eds. Central auditory assessment: the SSW test. San Diego: College Hill Press 1982;1–38.

21. Grimes AM, Grady CL, Foster NL, Sunderland T, Patronas NJ. Central auditory function in Alzheimer's disease. Neurology 1985;35:352–58.

22. Katz J. SSW Workshop Manual. Amherst, NY: Jack Katz 1979.

23. Broadbent D. The role of auditory localization in attention and memory span. J Exp Psych 1954;47:191–96.

24. Kimura D. Some effects of temporal-lobe damage on auditory perception. Can J Psych 1961;15:156–65.

25. Kimura D. Cerebral dominance and the perception of verbal stimuli. Can J Psych 1961;15:166–71.

26. Musiek FE. Assessment of central auditory dysfunction: the dichotic digit test revisited. Ear and Hearing 1983;4:79–83.

27. Berlin CI, McNeil MR. Dichotic listening. In: Lass NJ, ed. Issues in experimental phonetics. New York: Academic Press, 1976;327–87.

28. Cullen JK, Berlin CI, Hughes L, Thompson C, Samson D. Speech information flow: a model. In: Sullivan M, ed. Central auditory processing disorders. Omaha: University of Nebraska Medical Center, 1975;108–27.

29. Gelfand A, Silman S. Acoustic reflex thresholds in brain damaged subjects. Ear and Hearing 1982;3:93–95.

30. Cullen JK, Thompson CL. Masking release for subjects with temporal lobe resections. Arch Otolaryngol 1974;100:113–16.

31. Lynn GE, Gilroy J, Taylor PC, Leiser RP. Binaural masking level differences in neurological disorders. Arch Otolaryngol 1981;107:357–62.

32. Jerger JF, Brown D, Smith S. Effect of peripheral hearing loss on the masking level difference. Arch Otolaryngol 1984;110:290–96.

33. Keith RW. Interpretation of the Staggered Spondee Word (SSW) test. Ear and Hearing 1983;4:287–92.

34. Grimes AM, Grady CL, Foster NL, Sunderland T. Performance on the SSW in Alzheimer's disease. Paper presented at the annual meeting of the American Speech-Language-Hearing Association, Cincinnati, November 20, 1983.

35. Beck WG, Mueller HG, Sedgerk A. Measure of test-retest reliability of the SSW. SSW Reports 1985;7:8–11.

36. Jerger S. Decision matrix and information theory analyses in the evaluation of neuroaudiologic tests. Sem Hearing 1983;4:121–32.
37. Jerger S, Jerger JF. The evaluation of diagnostic audiometric tests. Audiology 1983;22:144–66.
38. Turner RG, Shepard NT, Frazer GH. Clincial performance of audiological and related diagnostic tests. Ear and Hearing 1984;5:187–94.

Chapter 12

Evoked Potentials and Head Injury in a Rehabilitation Setting

Maurice Rappaport

Evoked potential (EP) testing has become increasingly useful since the 1970s in rehabilitation settings. EP data contribute to the clinical assessment of a patient's disability by helping to identify sensory impairments as well as the extent and severity of central nervous system (CNS) dysfunction. Information obtained by X-rays or computed tomography (CT) scans shows structural rearrangements associated with trauma that may or may not reflect neurophysiologic impairments. In contrast, abnormal EPs directly indicate problems in neurophysiologic function. EP results have the power to monitor change in a patient's condition and can aid in predicting clinical outcome. Such information can be used to help decide on the needed frequency and intensity of rehabilitation efforts. In this context, EP results can contribute to the development of cost-effective rehabilitation care. Closely related to this consideration is the demonstrable capability of EP testing to assess sensory functioning in seriously head-injured, uncooperative patients. In certain instances, like impairment in visual acuity, EP testing can be used to help correct specific deficits.

EP ABNORMALITIES AND CLINICAL DISABILITY

It has been reported by a number of workers that EP pattern abnormalities are correlated with the clinical disability of the patient at the time of testing [1–8]. New findings, derived from tests on long-term head-injured patients, suggest that useful information on the overall disability of a patient can be obtained up to at least 18 mo after onset of injury. Rappaport et al [2] have demonstrated that the degree of abnormality of the EP pattern is not only related to the severity of patient disability but also the correlation increases from about .55 when one sensory modality is employed to about .78 when

189

three modalities (auditory, visual, and somatosensory) are used. These findings are supported by other workers [5–8]. It has been observed by several investigators that brain stem responses, in general, are less highly correlated with disability than cortical responses, at least among long-term survivors of traumatic brain injury. This becomes understandable when one realizes that survival usually implies that certain vegetative functions controlled or regulated by the brain stem (respiration, heart rate, blood pressure, etc.) have remained relatively intact; otherwise a patient probably would not have survived.

What disability factors are closely associated with multimodality EP abnormalities? By using the Disability Rating Scale [9], we identified arousability, awareness, and responsivity as reflected in the Glasgow Coma Scale (GCS); cognitive ability for self-care as reflected in the patient's ability to know when (but not necessarily be able) to feed, toilet, and groom himself; level of functioning in terms of degree of physical dependence or independence; and psychosocial adaptability in terms of ability to be employed productively either in a job, in the home, or in school. These factors appear to be closely associated with the results obtained from multimodality EP testing.

It should also be borne in mind that physical recovery, which is frequently the primary consideration in short stay acute care settings, may not be nearly as critical in the long term as cognitive recovery. Cognitive recovery takes much longer in severe head injury patients than physical recovery [10]. The challenge for long-term rehabilitation care is to be able to estimate the cognitive recovery potential. This would allow judgments to be made about the extent, intensity, and length of time that comprehensive but expensive rehabilitation efforts should be provided. EP testing can contribute to this assessment process as well as to predicting clinical outcome.

EP ABNORMALITIES AND CLINICAL OUTCOME

There is evidence that EP patterns have the power to predict ultimate clinical outcome. This power is limited by the current state of the art, but there may be ways to improve this predictability. Also, as reported by Anderson and co-workers [5], some EP patterns are reliable predictors of unfavorable outcomes only while others are predictive of both favorable and unfavorable outcomes. Brain stem auditory potentials (BAEPs) and visual evoked potentials (VEPs) fit into the former category, while somatosensory evoked potentials (SSEPs) fit into the latter. However, Rappaport et al found that each of the three modalities had some predictive power [2]. Although correlations between outcome and multimodality EP data were in the region of .40, they were significant. In contrast, a Fisher exact probability of .0004 was found between cortical AEP and VEP pattern abnormalities and clinical outcome in infants and young children involved in drownings [3]. Newlon and Greenberg [4] and Greenberg et al [7,8] have reported a relationship between degree of EP abnormality and both degree of clinical impairment and length of time to recovery after head injury. For example, they report that head injury patients with minimal EP abnormalities attain maximal recovery in about 3 mo, while those with severer EP abnormalities may take 6 to 12 mo to demonstrate maximal recovery, providing intensive rehabilitation takes place in the interim. Greenberg et al [8] have shown that EP patterns provide better predictability of specific sensory defects in head-injured patients than clinical judgment.

More recently it has been observed that EP patterns obtained from long-term severe head-injured patients a considerable time after injury (up to almost 1 yr afterward) can provide information on whether there are likely to be further changes in the patient's clinical condition. In Figure 12.1 are examples of such EP patterns. One set of VEP and SEP patterns from a 24-yr-old female (F24) obtained 10 mo after a motor vehicle accident appeared sufficiently robust that they suggested the patient would show reasonable progress if intensive rehabilitation efforts were continued. This patient went

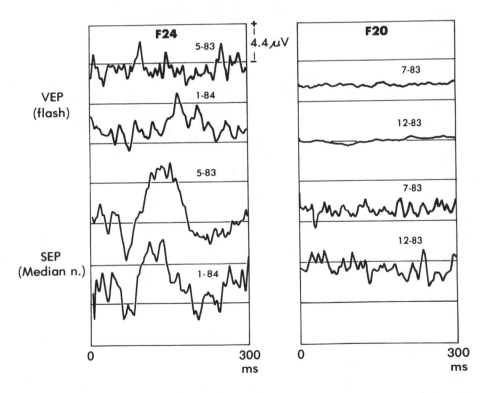

Figure 12.1   Visual (flash) and somatosensory (median nerve) evoked potential patterns for long-term patients with serious head injuries undergoing intensive rehabilitation. Relatively good patterns for F24 were associated with relatively good response to rehabilitation efforts. Poor patterns for F20 were associated with poor response to rehabilitation efforts.

from a disability rating (DR) of 21 (extremely severe disability) to a DR score of 13 (severe disability) 18 mo after date of injury to a DR score of 9 (moderately severe disability) about 24 mo after injury. Improvement in her clinical condition was reflected in an ability to communicate via a word board, to give clear signals about her need for toileting, and to give information on her need for food and wanting to groom herself.

Also in Figure 12.1 are examples of EP patterns obtained from a 20-yr-old female (F20) who suffered a respiratory arrest during a medical procedure 7 mo prior to her initial EP testing. This patient had a disability rating score of 27 (extreme vegetative state). The patterns were so poor and abnormal that it was felt that this patient would show little or no progress with the passage of time despite intensive rehabilitation efforts. When she was re-examined 5 mo later (approximately 1 yr after injury), no significant clinical change had been noted either in her EP patterns or in her clinical condition. When she was re-examined 19 mo after injury her DR score was still 27.

These two cases are examples of how EP patterns obtained a considerable time after brain injury provide important useful indications of a patient's current condition, ultimate outcome, and the likelihood of success of intensive rehabilitation care.

The scale one uses to measure outcome is an important consideration. The Glasgow Outcome Scale (GOS) is often used, and while its few outcome categories have utility, it is relatively insensitive to the types of changes seen in patients in long-term rehabilitation programs. For this purpose the Disability Rating Scale [9] appears more sensitive [2,11,12]. (A revised DR scale is currently being tested in an effort to increase sensitivity so that small changes in long-term head-injured patients can be more easily detected to facilitate rehabilitation planning in traumatic brain injury units.)

As mentioned, there may be ways of improving the sensitivity of EP testing to forecast outcome more accurately, particularly cognitive outcome. Up to now most EP testing has been aimed at primarily assessing neurophysiologic functioning. However, EP testing has the potential to assess neuropsychologic functioning, at least to a limited extent. This theoretical capability could be put to use to evaluate higher level cognitive functioning in head injury patients. One idea being explored in our laboratory is the use of EP testing in a conditioning paradigm. The approach consists of presenting the patient with two stimuli—one occurring with a high probability and the other with a low probability. Normal subjects who can attend are asked to count the number of low probability stimuli. This leads to the P300 phenomenon—i.e., the occurrence of a positive-going peak approximately 300 msec after the onset of the low probability stimulus. This is thought to reflect higher cortical activities associated with attention, perception, and discrimination, among other things. Obviously, seriously head-injured patients cannot be instructed to carry out this task. It should be possible, however, to determine if such patients are intact enough to establish at least a simple conditioned response. This, it would seem, should be achievable and testable by giving the patient a fairly high intensity somatosensory stimulation in association with the occurrence of a low probability signal like the presentation of a brief tone of a designated frequency. If, in a given patient, this leads to a conditioned P300 response, then it can be assumed that such a patient is in better condition and has sustained less brain damage than a patient who shows no such ability to establish a conditioned response. In this context it would be reasonable to anticipate and to predict that the former patient would ultimately show better long-term cognitive recovery than would the latter. In this way, or with some variation of this approach, it would appear reasonable to expect the power of prediction of outcome through EP testing to increase significantly.

SUMMARY

EP testing has application in rehabilitation programs, especially in the ability to help identify sensory and cognitive deficits in relatively nonresponsive head-injured patients. EP testing is currently being used to help assess clinical disability and outcome. EP results do have predictive power in terms of the ultimate degree of impairment and time to recovery. In the rehabilitation setting, they are useful in determining whether or not initiating or continuing rehabilitation efforts are likely to be worthwhile for a specific patient. We are exploring the role of using EPs to predict when specific therapeutic interventions should be initiated or terminated in severely brain-injured patients.

REFERENCES

1. Rappaport M, Hopkins HK, Hall K, Belleza T. Evoked potentials and head injury: 1. Rating of evoked potential abnormality. Clin Electroencephalog 1981;12:154–66.
2. Rappaport M, Hopkins HK, Hall K, Belleza T. Evoked potentials and head injury: 2. Clinical applications. Clin Electroencephalog 1981;12:167–76.
3. Rappaport M, Malony JR, Ortega H, Fetzer D, Hall K. Survival in young children after drowning: brain evoked potential patterns as outcome predictors. Clin Electroencephalog 1985.
4. Newlon PG, Greenberg RP. Assessment of brain function with multimodality evoked potentials. In: Rosenthal M, Griffith ER, Bond MR, Miller JD, eds. Rehabilitation of the head injured adult. Philadelphia: F.A. Davis, 1983;75–95.
5. Anderson D, Bundlie S, Rockswold GL. Multimodality evoked potentials in closed head trauma. Arch Neurol 1984;41:369–74.
6. Lindsay KW, Carlin J, Kennedy I, Fry J, McInnes A. Evoked potentials in severe head injury—analysis and relation to outcome. J Neurol Neurosurg Psychiatry 1981;44:796–802.
7. Greenberg RP, Mayer DJ, Becker DP, Miller JD. Evaluation of brain function in severe head trauma with multimodality evoked potentials. Part 1: evoked brain-injury potentials methods and analysis. J Neurosurg 1977;47:150–63.

8. Greenberg RP, Becker DP, Miller JP, Mayer DJ. Evaluation of brain function in severe human head trauma with multimodality evoked potentials. Part 2: Localization of brain dysfunction and correlation with posttraumatic neurological conditions. J Neurosurg 1977;47:163–77.

9. Rappaport M, Hall KM, Hopkins K, Belleza T. Disability rating scale for severe head trauma: coma to community. Arch Phys Med Rehabil 1982;63:118–23.

10. Mackworth NH, Mackworth JF, Cope DN. Towards an interpretation of head injury recovery trends. In: NIHR Report. Severe head trauma: a comprehensive medical approach. San Jose, Calif.: Institute for Medical Research, 1982; ch VIII, p 1–66.

11. Hall KM, Cope ND, Rappaport M. Glasgow Outcome Scale and Disability Rating Scale: comparative usefulness in following recovery in traumatic head injury. Arch Phys Med Rehabil 1985;66:35–37.

12. Eliason MR, Topp BW. Predictive validity of Rappaport's disability rating scale in subjects with acute brain dysfunction. Phys Ther 1984;64:1357–60.

Part III

Recovery and Outcome Issues

Harvey S. Levin

The chapters included in this part reflect the impressive progress made during the 1970s and early 1980s on characterizing the outcome of head injury. Information concerning outcome after head injury is essential for evaluating treatment efficacy, planning facilities for rehabilitation, and maintaining accurate epidemiologic data on this major public health problem. Despite the numerous contributions to the measurement of outcome, there remain unresolved methodological issues concerning the appropriate use and limitations of global categories of outcome, specific indexes of adjustment to daily activities, and neuropsychological measures.

Specific measures that are appropriate for assessing outcome at one point in the recovery process may not be optimal for other stages. Further, procedures and criteria for evaluating outcome in adults may require modification for use in children. There is continuing debate concerning the interval at which outcome of head injury should be assessed. Should the interval be uniform or varied according to which functions are under investigation? Should the interval vary with the severity of injury and the age of the patient?

Clinicians and investigators have also expressed concern about the so-called ecologic validity of outcome measures. Are laboratory tasks and interview schedules related to the head-injured patient's performance in real life situations? The issue of generalization across situations is important not only for measures of outcome but also for the effects of rehabilitation. The chapters in this part address many of these issues and raise additional questions for future research.

Chapter 13

Issues in the Evaluation of Rehabilitation Effects

Tessa Hart
Mary Ellen Hayden

Rehabilitation after head injury is expensive in terms of time, energy, and monetary resources. The cost has increased progressively over the last few years since the realization that for the majority of patients cognitive and behavioral limitations are more handicapping in the long run than physical or sensorimotor impairments [1]. Thus, many rehabilitation facilities have expanded their head trauma programs to include a heavy emphasis on the cognitive and behavioral deficits as well as on interventions for the family system. The efficacy of these new interventions, as well as that of some of the more traditional rehabilitation techniques, has not been unequivocally demonstrated. In addition, the offering of rehabilitation services to consumers implies a better prognosis than would be expected without treatment. Obviously, if functional outcome is not enhanced as a result of a treatment, the provision of that treatment raises serious ethical questions. It is, therefore, incumbent on rehabilitation specialists to obtain research data that show the efficacy or lack of efficacy of their treatment programs.

Baddeley, Meade, and Newcombe [2] point out that studies on rehabilitation should be both tractable (i.e., likely to yield valid data at reasonable cost) and "likely to lead to some practical outcome" (p. 138)—i.e., ecologically valid. The idea of tractability assumes that only interpretable and valid data are worth the considerable effort and expense involved in their collection. The design of a tractable study requires careful attention to factors such as spontaneous recovery, the selection of subjects, and the definition of what groups and settings are appropriate for generalization of the research results. These issues are discussed in the first section of this chapter.

The idea of ecological validity assumes that the most carefully designed study is of little practical value if it demonstrates change only on some measure irrelevant to the everyday functioning of the patient. We conclude with a discussion of this issue, with emphasis on the problems most relevant to the closed head injury population.

197

TRACTABILITY OF RESEARCH DESIGN

In their classic monograph on research design, which focused mainly on problems encountered in educational and psychological research, Campbell and Stanley identified internal and external validity as the major criteria by which to evaluate research designs and data [3]. Internal validity is "the basic minimum without which any experiment is uninterpretable: Did in fact the experimental treatments make a difference in this specific experimental instance?" (p. 5). The internal validity of a research design is the extent to which change in a dependent variable, or variables, may be attributed to a treatment or intervention rather than to extraneous factors. Once internal validity has been established, external validity may be evaluated. The issue of external validity is one of generalizability of the research results: "To what populations, settings, treatment variables, and measurement variables can this effect be generalized?" (p. 5). Campbell and Stanley discuss numerous threats to both types of validity encountered in social science research. We are particularly interested in those threats most likely to occur in research on the efficacy of rehabilitation and draw from the literature in this area to provide specific illustrations.

Internal Validity

In clinical settings, many factors that are difficult to control for practical or ethical reasons can undermine the interpretation of data. Probably the most common threats to internal validity are the effects of time, factors in the selection and assignment of subjects, and the effects of the evaluation. Placebo effects also warrant careful attention in any study of treatment effects.

Effects of Time

One of the most difficult problems facing any researcher interested in the efficacy of rehabilitation is separating the effects of treatment from improvements that occur naturally over the same time interval. Campbell and Stanley [3] discuss a set of time-dependent threats to internal validity, termed *maturation* effects, that include "spontaneous remission, analogous to wound healing, [that] may be mistaken for the specific effect of a remedial [treatment]" (p. 8). The recovery issue is particularly important in evaluating rehabilitation after head injury, since questions are now being raised about the previously hypothesized slowing of recovery after a brief period of time [4]. In studies that follow a single group of head trauma cases enrolled in a specific rehabilitation program, it is therefore difficult to separate the effects of treatment from those of natural long-term recovery [5].

The most desirable method of controlling for spontaneous recovery is to use comparable subjects who are randomly assigned to a no-treatment condition. This method should eliminate natural time-dependent change as an alternative explanation of improvement seen in the group assigned to treatment. However, if this method is to act as an adequate control, changes in the treatment and control groups should be evaluated at the same time. Otherwise, differences between the groups could be due to so-called *historical* factors. With respect to rehabilitation research, these factors could refer to any changes in policy or procedure on the unit or in the facility in which the research is conducted. If treatment and control groups are evaluated at different times, then historical factors could account for differences between groups apart from any genuine treatment effects.

Jellinek and Harvey wished to evaluate whether the presence of vocational/educational services would affect employment 2 to 3 yr post trauma [6]. They compared employment outcome for patients treated during 1977 (before the service was available) with that of a 1978 sample (after the addition of services). Although there was a significant increase in the rate of employment among patients treated in 1978, the fact that the comparison groups were observed and treated at different times complicates the interpretation of the results. Over a 2 yr period, many changes in hospital policy or procedure could have taken place concurrently with the addition of vocational/educational services. For example, admission criteria might have been modified such that patients accepted on the unit were more likely to be employable regardless of treatment. This factor may well have been operating in this particular case since of the forty-three subjects treated in 1977, only thirty were retrospectively judged to be appropriate for vocational/educational services. In 1978, however, all forty-three patients were deemed appropriate. Thus, the increase in employment rates cannot confidently be attributed to any one factor, including the one targeted in the study. In this type of research design, the confounding factors may be undetectable through retrospective analysis. For example, over a period of months or years, even a subtle increase in the overall level of staff expertise and sophistication could account for significant changes in rehabilitation outcome.

Another method of controlling for the effects of spontaneous recovery, which does not require the use of a control group, is to evaluate the fit of observed data to models of recovery and treatment generated a priori. Hart, Carbonari, and Sheer used this technique in a multiple-single-case design, with right hemisphere stroke patients undergoing trials of cognitive remediation [7]. Observed changes in scores on a psychometric battery and on selected activities of daily living were used as dependent measures in a multiple regression, where the independent variables were coded vectors modeling pure recovery and pure treatment. While both models predicted that the scores would improve over time (a 4 wk period), the shape of the vectors was different because the intervention did not begin until the third week of the observation period. Thus, the recovery model predicted linear improvement from week to week, while the treatment model predicted an abrupt shift after 2 wk of observation. The regression analysis was used to estimate the proportion of variance in the observed scores due uniquely to treatment, uniquely to recovery, and to their shared effect. With this procedure, it is important that the recovery and treatment models be statistically separable (although they cannot be independent) to estimate the relative contribution of each process to observed changes in the dependent variable.

Treatment models are fairly easy to define because the form, magnitude, and duration of the intervention are under the experimenter's control. Recovery, however, must be modeled based on our current knowledge of pathologic processes that differ on etiology, severity, and many other parameters. Much more insight into the natural history of head trauma and other types of central nervous system (CNS) insult is needed so we can generate appropriate models against which to evaluate treatment effects. The issue becomes even more complex with the growing evidence that different aspects of cognitive and behavioral function recover at different rates [8].

Selection and Assignment of Subjects

A true experimental design [3] must include random assignment of the available pool of subjects so that the groups may be considered initially equivalent. In a clinical setting, randomly assigning patients to a no-treatment condition presents enormous practical and ethical problems. These difficulties would appear to be greater for broad research questions. Consider the case of an experimenter who wonders if a 6 mo stay on his or her rehabilitation unit leads to better functional outcome than no treatment at all. It would be impossible to answer this question by randomly assigning half of the appropriate subjects to 6 mo of inactivity. Random assignment is feasible, however, in clinical studies that undertake a finer grained analysis of treatment effects. For example, the question of whether speech therapy method A or method B causes greater functional improvement in dysarthric patients after 3 mo is amenable to random assignment if there is no reason to believe that either method is really equivalent to withholding treatment. An experimental intervention may also be contrasted with routine or standard treatment [9]. Thus, one answer to the random assignment dilemma is to begin with more specific research questions, focusing on particular types or aspects of intervention rather than on the global variable, treatment.

Another way to circumvent the problems associated with random assignment of subjects is to assign treatments randomly to preexisting, indivisible groups. Campbell and Stanley refer to this as the "nonequivalent control group design," illustrated in the educational literature by the practice of randomly assigning teaching methods or curricula to classrooms of pupils [3]. A comparable procedure in a rehabilitation setting might be to choose units or floors housing similar patients and randomly assign different experimental unitwide interventions. For example, one floor of posttraumatic patients could receive orientation therapy through special classes held once or twice each day, while another unit of patients drawn from the same population could experience more of an orientation milieu with visual cues in every room, verbal reminders from nurses, etc. As described by Campbell and Stanley, this design includes a pretest on the dependent variable to estimate the pretreatment equivalence of the groups.

The nonequivalent control group design should not be confused with what Campbell and Stanley call the "static group comparison" [3]. In the latter design, instead of randomly assigning treatments to equivalent groups of patients, the researcher compares groups who have been preselected for reasons beyond his or her control. For example, patients who have undergone a course of treatment might be compared to a group with similar diagnoses who were unable or unwilling to participate in therapy. The obvious difficulty with this design is that even if the groups differ on the dependent variable after treatment, the effects of intervention can never be disentangled from the effects of preexisting differences, both known and unknown.

An example of a static group comparison is provided by Prigatano et al [10], who described an intensive 6 mo treatment program for postacute closed head injury patients. Pre to post changes on measures of neuropsychological and psychological functioning were compared to 6 mo changes in the scores of a "control group" of head trauma patients who had been re-evaluated at the appropriate interval. Some of these control subjects had been recommended for the treatment program, but "for a variety of reasons, these recommendations were not followed" (p. 507). In any use of this type of control group (as with the use of nonattendees as controls in psychotherapy outcome research), the researcher cannot know whether significant findings are an artifact of treating an extraordinarily motivated group, one which might have improved to an unusual degree without any treatment. Even if motivation could be ruled out as an extraneous factor, other contaminating variables may be postulated. If a patient attends therapy because he is able to pay for it or because of pressure from his family, this could indicate a home environment more favorable for recovery (with or without treatment) than if the family is passive or disinterested.

A common practice, carried out in an attempt to increase the pretreatment equivalence of subjects who cannot be randomly assigned, is matching on some variable or variables assumed to affect performance on the dependent measure. Prigatano et al [10], e.g., attempted to choose controls who matched program participants on variables such as age, injury severity, and neurologic sequelae. Campbell and Stanley caution that matching subjects in a static group comparison is an ineffective and potentially misleading control for the pretreatment nonequivalence of groups [3]. In some cases, matching can ensure that the groups are not equivalent on some important variable. For example, Cope and Hall attempted to determine whether head trauma victims admitted to a rehabilitation unit early (within 35 day post injury) would enjoy a shorter hospital stay and better functional recovery than those admitted late (after 35 day) [11]. Since their sample of early admissions had a coma duration of fewer than 15 day, Cope and Hall retrospectively matched to them a sample of late-admitted patients who had also had coma of 2 wk or less. Unfortunately, this procedure probably ensured that the patients admitted for rehabilitation later must have suffered complicating factors other than protracted coma that precluded their early admission to a rehabilitation unit (e.g., a prolonged state of agitation). Thus, it is no surprise that the early group showed less psychological impairment, less incontinence, and fewer bilateral cerebral lesions. It is also no surprise that the late group remained hospitalized for twice as long—one of the main findings attributed to late admission.

One alternative to the hazards of matching is the procedure known as blocking: pairing subjects on a variable of interest, then randomly assigning one member of each pair to different treatment conditions. This type of design was used by Relander, Troupp, and Bjorkesten, who grouped subjects with mild head injuries according to age, sex, type of insurance, and the length of posttraumatic amnesia [12]. Subjects within these matched groups were randomly assigned either to routine treatment or to an active schedule that emphasized early activity, physiotherapy, and participation in follow-up clinics. The active group missed significantly less time from work although they spent about the same amount of total time in the hospital.

A final issue important for subject selection involves the statistical phenomenon of regression toward the mean [3]. Simply stated, individuals who obtain extreme scores on an initial measurement of some variable will tend to score closer to the population mean on a subsequent measurement. Thus, e.g., patients recruited for a study on cognitive retraining because of their low scores on a psychometric test may appear to improve over time because their second test scores tend to be higher. The obvious control for statistical regression is the use of a comparison group with equally extreme scores on initial testing (e.g., [9]). This allows the researcher to separate the effects of regression from the effects of treatment when interpreting different scores for groups with initial scores that deviate significantly from the population mean.

Effects of Testing

Another threat that is of particular concern in rehabilitation settings is the potentially confounding effects of the number of observations necessary to detect change. If the same test instrument is used before and after intervention, it is possible that higher scores could reflect practice effects rather than treatment effects. Different types of assessment methods may be expected to show different degrees of test-retest improvement. Indexes of sensorimotor function, like those found on a standard neurologic examination, would be of less concern in this regard than measures of higher cognitive functions.

For example, the psychological and neuropsychological literature contains considerable discussion of practice effects on the Wechsler Adult Intelligence Scale (WAIS). Matarazzo, Carmody, and Jacobs reviewed a group of studies using subjects ranging in age from 19 to 70 yr with test-retest intervals from 1 wk to over 10 yr [13]. They found a mean test-retest increase of 5 IQ points. Based on their data, they suggested that improvement should be on the order of 15 points to be interpreted as an effect of something other than practice. However, Shatz took exception to the use of this rule when dealing with brain-injured individuals [14]. He cited a study by Kendrick and Post, who found that elderly depressed patients showed a reliable practice effect on the WAIS whereas those with organic brain syndrome did not [15]. Dodrill and Troupin found that younger patients suffering from major seizure disorders showed IQ losses on WAIS posttesting at 6 and 12 mo follow-up [16]. No significant improvements from baseline testing were found until the fourth administration of the WAIS, between 18 and 29 mo post baseline. Practice effects are similarly weak in patients with carotid artery disease [17]. Based on these and other studies, Shatz concluded that for subjects with known cerebral dysfunction, pre-to-posttest improvement on the WAIS could be confidently attributed to recovery or treatment effects. There is no simple solution to this problem, particularly since practice effects in brain-injured subjects have not been investigated extensively for measures of higher cognitive function other than the WAIS. One possible solution is to use alternate forms of the measurement instrument at different test intervals [18].

A subject's reaction to the measurement process may also be a testing effect that threatens internal validity. It has long been recognized in the social sciences that certain measures are more reactive (i.e., capable of causing behavior change) than others that serve as relatively passive records of behavior. The classic example cited by Campbell and Stanley is the initial weigh-in on a weight control program, which might alone be an impetus to weight reduction [3]. In a rehabilitation setting, an assessment technique could prove reactive if it brings the types or degrees of deficits forcefully to the subject's attention. The effects of intervention targeted at the deficit area could then be difficult to disentangle from the subject's efforts to improve his or her later standing on the assessment measure.

Another testing issue raised by Campbell and Stanley is one they call "instrumentation," referring to changes in the measurement instrument between the pretest and the posttest [3]. In rehabilitation research, the most likely manifestation of this problem would be changes in the observers or testers who are measuring treatment effects. Becoming familiar with a test battery or observational measure over the course of a research project could lead an evaluator to adopt different criteria for scoring or interpretation, albeit at an unconscious level. More obvious instrumentation problems may occur if the pre- and posttests are administered by different people. Therefore, instrumentation is less of a threat to validity the more objective and standardized is the assessment procedure.

To some extent, the threats to internal validity associated with testing factors can be circumvented by choosing designs that do not require a pretest and/or by using appropriate control groups who undergo testing at the same intervals as the experimental group. In studies using control groups, it is important to ensure that all subjects are assessed by the same evaluators (or by randomly assigned evaluators). Ideally, the people who measure the outcome of rehabilitative treatments should be blind to the experimental status of the subjects, although this is difficult to achieve in most clinical settings.

Placebo Effects

Any change in behavior or outcome that is associated with a program of treatment but is not related specifically to the treatment may be considered a placebo effect. While these nonspecific effects are of interest in their own right, they also confound results by helping to obscure the relationships among specific treatment variables and outcome variables. Researchers interested in the effects of rehabilitation must recognize the problem of extricating the influences of treatment from "the effect of being cared for by a dedicated team" [19, p. 1035]. There are also nonspecific effects, both positive and negative, associated with participation in a novel or unusual therapeutic program. The ideal control for placebo effects is a sham treatment condition with credibility equal to that of the true intervention [20]. Sham treatments are easier to accomplish when the interventions are unusual (i.e., not widely recognized by laypersons) or targeted toward a narrow spectrum of behavior. For example, in the study by Hart and co-workers [7], the treatment consisted of repeated practice on microcomputer programs for remediation of left neglect or constructional dyspraxia [21]. Prior to intervention, subjects participated in a sham treatment (baseline) phase in which the computer activities were designed to have minimal impact on these cognitive functions. However, compared to the actual treatment phase, the baseline phase provided equal time on the computer (a novel medium for most subjects) and equal encouragement and reinforcement from the therapist.

External Validity

Given that a program of research has been developed and executed with careful attention to factors that affect internal validity, and given that an effect of the treatment has been established, the developer (or consumer) of research still must also consider the degree to which these results may be applied in other situations. An experimental treatment that works in one facility may have no apparent effect in another, for a variety of reasons related to the setting, the type of treatment offered, and the patient population chosen for study.

The effects of the setting on the external validity of research can be subtle. The cumulative effect of even slight differences in the implementation of a rehabilitation program or technique could be significant, in either a positive or negative direction. Attempts to generalize research findings across settings could also be compromised by "multiple-treatment interference" [3]. This refers to the possibility that any experimental treatment X is effective only in combination with a prior treatment Y. Thus, treatment X would appear to work only in settings or programs that incorporate treatment Y. As a hypothetical example, a program of electromyogram (EMG) biofeedback training might prove successful for remediating hemiplegia only in facilities that offer a certain type of muscle-strengthening program as part of their standard treatment.

A second potential threat to external validity concerns the procedures used to sample from the population of interest. Generalization of research results to a wider population (e.g., a diagnostic group) becomes tenuous if a small or unrepresentative sample is used [22]. An unrepresentative sample could result from overstrict inclusion criteria such that the treatment is tested on a relatively select group of patients. For example, a remediation proven effective in a group of healthy, alert stroke patients may or may not be expected to generalize to stroke patients with other serious medical problems. Sample selection problems may also occur with the closed head injury population because the risk of head trauma covaries with subject attributes commonly used as exclusion criteria for research. In the experience of one prominent investigator, "about 20% of adult hospital admissions for head injury are unsuitable for investigation . . . because of previous conditions including psychiatric disorder, alcohol/drug abuse, and mental subnormality" [23, p. 58]. While there are sound reasons for controlling such factors when investigating specific relationships between brain injury and behavior, the question remains whether the effect of therapeutic programs will extend to the sizable minority of patients with these premorbid characteristics.

A related question concerns the extent to which the results of rehabilitation research may be generalized from one patient population to another. It has been our experience that interventions that are successful for one more or less homogeneous group (e.g., right hemisphere stroke patients) may be applied to a different group (e.g., head-injured patients) only with extensive modifications that take into account the basic underlying differences in cognitive dysfunction. Even very circumscribed remediation procedures, like the use of cueing systems to facilitate verbal list learning, show dramatically different degrees of effectiveness depending on the underlying nature of the verbal memory deficit [24,25].

In the psychology literature, the concept of external validity has taken on meaning in addition to the issues of generalizability across settings and patient populations. The term is frequently used to denote the fidelity of an experimental procedure to real world, everyday functions or activities. We agree with Berkowitz and Donnerstein [26] that the so-called ecological validity [27] of an experiment is profitably examined separately from its external validity. In research on rehabilitation, ecological validity is of particular concern when psychometric measures are used to assess outcome and thereby to predict the ability to function in the real world. The next section uses case material to support the idea that standard neuropsychological tests may have limited ecological validity when they are used as outcome measures for rehabilitation after closed head injury.

Ecological Validity

Most psychological and neuropsychological assessment techniques were developed for diagnostic purposes. Relatively little attention has been paid to their value for predicting the ability to resume work, drive a car, or participate in a normal range of social activities [28–30]. The criteria used to validate traditional neuropsychological tests, such as locus of lesion or diagnostic category, are therefore quite different from the more functional outcome criteria of interest to most researchers in the field of rehabilitation. Considering the current lack of data correlating neuropsychological test results with measures of everyday functioning, ecological validity is compromised in any study using only psychometric outcome measures.

As a consequence of the cognitive sequelae of closed head injury, the functional relevance of psychometric test scores is even more tenuous in this population than in other patient groups. The pathophysiology of head trauma is consistent with a basic underlying deficit in information processing on which may be superimposed specific deficits referable to focal lesions [31]. Patients with information-processing limitations may be expected to show disproportionate decrements in performance when faced with increased informational complexity, distraction, or stress [32]. Therefore, their ability to perform a task in a highly structured, quiet, one-on-one testing situation may not be at all reflective of their ability to perform a similar task in a less structured, more distracting, informationally complex environment. A psychometric approach to research on head trauma could be very misleading if generalizations to environmentally relevant activities are desired. Clinicians experienced with head injury are painfully aware that many of these patients function essentially within normal limits on many formal neuropsychological tests and then show significant difficulties at work, in social situations, or at school. Past tendencies to attribute these dysfunctions to personality problems have, for the most part, given way to an understanding that the informational complexity of a structured test setting is significantly different from that of most real world situations. Thus, scores on a standardized neuropsychological battery may grossly overestimate a patient's ability to function in everyday life.

A second factor that can affect the ecological relevance of neuropsychological test scores involves the extent to which an individual has learned to compensate for his or her cognitive deficits by using strategies or crutches in daily life. These compensatory techniques may not be applied in the test situation, in which case the psychometric data may grossly underestimate everyday functioning.

These points are illustrated by the case material presented in Table 13.1. The table shows selected neuropsychological test scores for two patients (RE and MT) who had suffered severe closed head injuries. Both patients had WAIS-R IQ scores in the average range. Immediate auditory memory (digit span) was also intact. On more demanding tests of memory, however, they performed quite differently. RE had significantly more difficulty than MT in

Table 13.1 Selected Neuropsychological Test Scores

Test	RE	MT
WAIS-R		
Full Scale IQ	100	91
Verbal IQ	98	91
Performance IQ	104	93
Memory tests		
Digit span		
Forward	6	9
Backward	5	4
Scaled score	10	12
Buschke Selective Reminding		
Procedure [33]		
Long-term retrieval (%ile)	0	10
Long-term store (%ile)	0	16
Consistent long-term retrieval (%ile)	0	0
30 min recall (no. words/12)	2	0
Wechsler Memory Scale, Logical		
Memory (Story A)		
Scale Score [34]	6	13
Continuous Recognition Memory [35]		
Hits (%ile)	9	38
False alarms (%ile)	2	21
Total (%ile)	2	77

relating the elements of a prose passage (Wechsler Memory Scale, Logical Memory) and identifying recurring items in a series of perceptually similar pictures (Continuous Recognition Memory). On both these measures, MT's scores were entirely within normal limits. Both patients had difficulty on a sensitive measure of verbal learning (Buschke Selective Reminding Procedure), although here again RE's deficits were more profound.

On other neuropsychological tests not shown in Table 13.1, both patients demonstrated normal somatosensory, visual-perceptual, and linguistic function. MT's motor function scores were within normal limits, but RE demonstrated motor disinhibition and impairments of speed and dexterity.

The results of formal neuropsychological testing for MT suggested intact cognitive function, except for difficulty with consistent retrieval and delayed recall of verbal material. RE, in contrast, displayed profound memory impairments across the board, as well as some motor deficits. Conventional wisdom would predict that MT's social and vocational adjustment would be superior by virtue of his superior neuropsychological test performance. Soon after the evaluations shown in Table 13.1, both MT and RE were placed in full-time therapeutic work trials monitored by trained observers on site. The outcome of these trials provided a striking contrast: RE completed 5 mo on the job with excellent supervisor's ratings and was offered a permanent paid position based on his performance. MT was discharged from his work trial on the second day. He had become acutely confused and disoriented, and his performance was so poor that it was disruptive to other workers.

The predictive failure of the neuropsychological battery in this case may be understood in light of the preceding points on ecological validity. RE's functional capacity was grossly underestimated by the psychometric assessment. Just prior to testing, RE had completed a full-time, 6 mo program for cognitive, interpersonal, and vocational rehabilitation. The goal of the program was to compensate for the typical effects of head injury by helping patients to maintain cognitive efficiency in the face of progressively greater informational complexity and to learn compensatory strategies for residual cognitive deficits. Thus, RE had already received training in situations that gradually approximated naturalistic information-processing demands. In addition, he was given extensive practice in the consistent use of strategies to compensate for the severe memory impairments. Throughout the 5 mo of his work trial, RE was observed to use these compensations very effectively. His vocational potential was underestimated by the results of formal testing because the strategies he had learned were neither applicable nor relevant to psychometric measures of memory function.

The test results for MT, in contrast, appeared to overestimate his ability to function in a setting more informationally complex than the assessment situation. Prior to his evaluation, MT had had none of the formal training received by RE, although he had participated in a program of cognitive retraining for specific deficits. As a final note to this case presentation, MT was eventually treated in a program similar to RE's. He successfully completed a second work trial and is now competitively employed.

These cases underscore the dangers that can occur in predicting from test scores obtained under conditions of low information-processing requirements to situations in which factors such as complexity, stress, distraction, and fatigue are uncontrolled. Particularly in cases of severe head injury, which manifest almost universal information-processing deficits, measures of rehabilitation outcome should be taken in complex environments that approximate daily experience as closely as possible. Of course, such measures would be difficult to achieve both logistically and from the viewpoint of maintaining adequate experimental control. Baddeley, Meade, and Newcombe stress the need for objective measures of a patient's ability to function in everyday life [2]. The development of ecologically valid assessment tools is certainly one of the most pressing needs in the field of rehabilitation research.

SUMMARY

To summarize some important points from the preceding discussion, we believe that future studies in this area should attempt to accomplish the following:

1. Formulate research questions more specific than the all-encompassing, Is rehabilitation effective? More focused questions would have two clear advantages. First, investigations that compare, e.g., two different forms of a specific treatment lend themselves easily to a design in which homogeneous subjects are assigned at random to participation in one of the treatment groups. The pitfalls of designs that do not use random assignment and the ethical problems of withholding treatment may thus be avoided. Second, attempts to answer specific questions abut rehabilitation practices will help us to determine which aspects of a treatment method are responsible for observed changes and to refine our treatments for maximal efficiency.

2. Use homogeneous samples of brain-injured subjects in initial investigations, and cross validate research on different patient populations. Demonstrating a technique's effectiveness in certain populations (e.g., severe head injury) is an important first step. However, determining whether the same technique works for mild head injury or left hemisphere stroke is also of considerable theoretical and practical interest. Ideally, we will accumulate general principles allowing modification of a technique to fit a specific target population. Until then, studies using mixed groups of brain-damaged subjects are to be avoided unless results are reported separately for the different diagnostic groups in the sample.

3. Develop outcome measures that are tied as closely as possible to the real world behavior(s) of interest to the investigation. For example, some creative uses of questionnaire [36,37] and observational [38] methods for assessing memory have appeared in the neuropsychology literature. Although experimental measures may be expected to bring new methodological problems to bear, it is worth exploring their use to supplement or replace psychometric measures as outcome criteria [29].

4. Adopt new paradigms developed and/or advanced by clinical fields with similar research concerns. For example, many of the issues facing rehabilitation researchers have already been tackled by workers in the field of psychotherapy outcome research. The techniques of meta-analysis, in which the results of many reports in the literature are pooled to yield estimates of overall effectiveness and effect size, may be particularly applicable [39,40].

This chapter has presented some of the major concerns that should be addressed in the design or interpretation of any program of research on the effects of rehabilitation. We recognize fully the problems encountered in attempting to develop a valid research protocol in a clinical setting. Nevertheless, practical and theoretical advances in this field cannot occur without research that is internally valid, capable of replication and application in other settings, and meaningful in terms of everyday life.

Kazdin specified two criteria for evaluating treatment effects in clinical outcome studies: the experimental and the therapeutic [41]. Although he was referring to single-case designs, the distinction is relevant here. The experimental criterion—Did the treatment cause change?—is the question of internal validity. The therapeutic criterion—Did the treatment enhance the life of the patient?—is a very different, and more difficult, question. As difficult as it may be, every attempt to answer it will make us more responsive to the concerns of the patients in our care.

REFERENCES

1. Thomsen IV. Late outcome of very severe blunt head trauma: A 10–15 year second follow-up. J Neurol Neurosurg Psychiat 1984;47:260–68.
2. Baddeley A, Meade T, Newcombe F. Design problems in research on rehabilitation after brain damage. Int Rehab Med 1980;2:138–42.
3. Campbell DT, Stanley JC. Experimental and quasi-experimental designs for research. Chicago: Rand McNally and Co., 1966.
4. Dikmen S, Reitan RM, Temkin NR. Neuropsychological recovery in head injury. Arch Neurol 1983;40:333–38.
5. Najenson T, Mendelson L, Schechter I, David C, Mintz N, Groswasser Z. Rehabilitation after severe head injury. Scand J Rehab Med 1974;6:5–14.
6. Jellinek HM, Harvey RF. Vocational/educational services in a medical rehabilitation facility: Outcomes in spinal cord and brain injured patients. Arch Phys Med Rehab 1982;63:87–88.
7. Hart T, Carbonari JP, Sheer DE. A new single-case methodology for the evaluation of cognitive remediation techniques. Paper presented at the annual meeting of the International Neuropsychological Society, Houston, 1984.
8. Hier DB, Mondlock J, Caplan LR. Recovery of behavioral abnormalities after right hemisphere stroke. Neurology 1983;33:345–50.
9. Weinberg J, Diller L, Gordon WA, Gerstman LJ, Lieberman A, Lakin P, Hodges G, Ezrachi O. Visual scanning training effect on reading-related tasks in acquired right brain damage. Arch Phys Med Rehab 1977;58:479–86.
10. Prigatano GP, Fordyce DJ, Zeiner HK, Roueche JR, Pepping M, Wood BC. Neuropsychological rehabilitation after closed head injury in young adults. J Neurol Neurosurg Psychiat 1984;47:505–13.
11. Cope DN, Hall K. Head injury rehabilitation: Benefit of early intervention. Arch Phys Med Rehab 1982;63:433–37.
12. Relander M, Troupp H, Bjorkestan G. Controlled trial of treatment for cerebral concussion. Brit Med J 1972;4:777–79.
13. Matarazzo JD, Carmody TP, Jacobs LD. Test-retest reliability and stability of the WAIS: a literature review with implications for clinical practice. J Clin Neuropsychol 1980;2:89–105.
14. Shatz MW. WAIS practice effects in clinical neuropsychology. J Clin Neuropsychol 1981;3:171–79.
15. Kendrick DC, Post F. Differences in cognitive status between healthy, psychiatrically ill, and diffusely brain-damaged elderly subjects. Brit J Psychiat 1967;113:75–81.
16. Dodrill CB, Troupin AS. Effects of repeated administrations of a comprehensive neuropsychological battery among chronic epileptics. J Nerv Ment Dis 1975;161:185–90.

17. Duke R, Bloor B, Nugent R, Majzoub H. Changes in performance on WAIS, Trial Making Test and Finger Tapping Test associated with carotid artery surgery. Percept Motor Skills 1968;26:399–404.
18. Hannay HJ, Levin HS. Selective reminding test: an examination of the equivalence of four forms. J Clin Exp Neuropsychol 1985;7:251–63.
19. Medical Research Council. Research aspects of rehabilitation after acute brain damage in adults. Lancet 1982;2:1034–36.
20. Prokop CK, Bradley LA. Methodological issues in medical psychology and behavioral medicine research. In: Prokop CK, Bradley LA, eds. Medical psychology: contributions to behavioral medicine. New York: Academic Press, 1981;485–96.
21. Sheer DE. Programs I (attention training) and II (visual perceptual training) for cognitive remediation using the Apple II microcomputer. Unpublished software. Department of Psychology, University of Houston, Texas, 1982.
22. Mahoney MJ. Experimental methods and outcome evaluation. J Consult Clin Psychol 1978;46:660–72.
23. Levin HS, Benton AL, Grossman RG. Neurobehavioral consequences of closed head injury. New York: Oxford University Press, 1982.
24. Crovitz H. Memory retraining in brain-damaged patients: The airplane list. Cortex 1979;15:131–34.
25. Patten BM. The ancient art of memory: Usefulness in treatment. Arch Neurol 1972;26:25–31.
26. Berkowitz L, Donnerstein E. External validity is more than skin deep. Amer Psychol 1981;37:245–57.
27. Brunswik E. Representative design and probabilistic theory in a functional psychology. Psych Rev 1955;62:193–217.
28. Heaton RK, Pendleton MG. Use of neuropsychological tests to predict adult patients' everyday functioning. J Consult Clin Psychol 1981;49:807–21.
29. Hart T, Hayden ME. The ecological validity of neuropsychological assessment and remediation. In: Uzzell BP, Gross Y, eds. Clinical neuropsychology of intervention. Hingham, MA: Kluwer, in press.
30. Acker MB. Relationships between test scores and everyday life functioning. In: Uzzell BP, Gross Y, eds. Clinical neuropsychology of intervention. Hingham, MA: Kluwer, in press.
31. Hayden ME, Hart T. Rehabilitation of cognitive and behavioral dysfunction in head injury. In: Peterson LG, O'Shanick GJ, eds. Psychosomatic aspects of trauma. Basel: S. Karger, in press.
32. Gronwall D, Sampson H. The psychological effects of concussion. Auckland: Auckland University Press, 1974.
33. Buschke H, Fuld PA. Evaluating storage, retention, and retrieval in disordered memory and learning. Neurology 1974;24:1019–25.
34. Osborne D, Davis LJ. Standard scores for Wechsler Memory Scale subtests. J Clin Psychol 1978;34:115–16.
35. Hannay HJ, Levin HS, Grossman RG. Impaired recognition memory after head injury. Cortex 1979;15:269–83.
36. Sunderland A, Harris JE, Baddeley AD. Do laboratory tests predict everyday memory? A neuropsychological study. J Verb Learn Verb Behav 1983;22:341–57.
37. Sunderland A, Harris JE, Baddeley AD. Assessing everyday memory after severe head injury. In: Harris JE, Morris PE, eds. Everyday memory, actions and absent-mindedness. London: Academic Press, 1984;191–206.

38. Knight RG, Godfrey HPD. Reliability and validity of a scale for rating memory impairment in hospitalized amnesiacs. J Consult Clin Psychol 1984;52:769–73.
39. Green BF, Hall JA. Quantitative methods for literature reviews. Ann Rev Psychol 1984;35:37–53.
40. Landman JT, Dawes RM. Psychotherapy outcome. Am Psychol 1982;37:504–16.
41. Kazdin AE. Drawing valid inferences from case studies. J Consult Clin Psychol 1981;49:183–92.

Chapter 14

Sociological Parameters Affecting Comparisons of Long-term Outcome

Karen A. Wagner

In the United States the number of survivors of traumatic brain injury who have been hospitalized approaches 500,000 annually [1]. Their outcome depends not only on how they recover from their injury but also on the way the outcome is measured. The common parameter of most definitions of outcome is reference to the adequacy with which an individual resumes his premorbid lifestyle. Research on the eventual outcome of these patients is significant for medical practitioners, for the injured individuals and their families, and for society [2].

The point of view discussed in regard to these traumatically brain injured patients may be somewhat iconoclastic because the impact of the injury on the community at large is addressed rather than the impact of the injury on the individual [3,4,5]. To study the impact of injury on the community, a number of questions need to be reviewed. The effect of injury on the individual far exceeds the damage done to the brain tissue, but to what extent? Is only a special subset of individuals affected by brain trauma, and what effect does this problem have on the community? How long does it take these individuals to reintegrate into the society from which they came and resume a role within the community? Does the role that the traumatically brain-injured person resumes differ significantly from the previous role such that others change their roles to fill the gaps, creating a sort of domino effect?

When an individual's brain is injured and he is removed from society for a period of time, several things happen. The individual undergoes changes in his capabilities because of the damage to the brain and the extent to which rehabilitation is able to facilitate complete or partial recovery of function. The individual's place in society is somehow filled during the time he is hospitalized. The roles may not be filled as well as when the individual filled them, but the primary and most demanding tasks are done and life goes on. The community continues to grow, develop, and change. The impact of the national economy

213

on the community persists. Children mature and human emotions change. Companies expand or go bankrupt. Inflation rises or falls.

Because life goes on and change is constant, when the individual is deemed able to attempt to reintegrate into the world, he finds both himself and his community changed. As individuals vary, so do communities. Some communities provide a better milieu into which a patient can reintegrate. Some communities contain more individuals with characteristics known to be typical of a successful outcome. These individual and community differences are critical in the evaluation of the outcome of individuals following any injury but are particularly important in traumatic brain injury.

This chapter highlights the sociological differences that exist in different geographical areas. When comparing data from various long-term studies, these sociological parameters may account for some of the differences in outcome results. Clearly, these differences must be taken into account when attempting to generalize data reported in the literature to one's own patient population.

The sociological parameters often considered when assessing outcome from traumatic brain injury cannot be generalized in the same way that one would generalize physiological parameters. It is reasonable to assume that the normal range for intracranial pressure can be generalized from the United Kingdom to the USSR. However, the employability of an individual in Topeka, Kansas, versus that in Glasgow, Scotland, can be dramatically different. Yet, data on the sociological characteristics of the traumatic brain injured are generalized with the same assumed precision as the physiological characteristics.

The three sociological parameters that are assessed are education level, marital status, and employment. These parameters vary significantly in parts of the United States alone. Sociological data on three U.S. cities from which outcome studies on head injury have been reported are used: Charlottesville, Virginia; Houston, Texas; and San Diego, California. The variability is highly significant, and the differences between patient outcomes cannot be attributed to degree of severity, specific treatment modalities, or interventions without due consideration of the differences between the communities in which the patients live.

EDUCATION LEVEL

The amount of formal education one has completed can be taken as a gross index of mental capacity. An individual's results on a given psychological achievement/intelligence test can be influenced by the extent to which the individual progressed in school. A specific education level is often considered a prerequisite for employment in many jobs in the United States. Therefore, in a sense, one's education level contributes to who an individual is and his role within society.

In a 15 yr follow-up study by Dresser et al of 864 Korean conflict veterans, it was found that the single most important factor in predicting the probability of employment following head injury was the pre-injury mental status as evidenced by the Armed Forces Qualifications Test [6].

In a retrospective study of seventy-five brain-injured patients on a physical medicine and rehabilitation unit in California, Tobis et al reported that far fewer of these patients had returned to work than expected [7], when compared with other reports in the literature. They noted that the average number of years of eduction achieved by students of Orange County, California, was 12.2 to 12.4 yr, and in their study population it was 10.28. This is one of the few articles that makes a comparative analysis regarding the education level of their study subjects.

In the articles by Jane et al [8] and Rimel et al [9] on the outcome of head-injured patients in the full spectrum of severity, there is report of the education levels of the research population. In the moderate group, 42% had completed secondary education and 12% had completed 4 or more yr of college. In the mild group, 45% had completed secondary education and 17% had completed 4 or more yr of college. The article confirms the importance of pre-injury education level, especially in the mild group where the relation between education level and return to work 3 mo after injury was significant at the p = .001 level. They make no mention of the education level of the community at large; thus, the reader has no basis for comparison.

In the 2 yr prospective follow-up study conducted at the Division of Neurosurgery, University of Texas Medical School at Houston, between 1980 and 1982, the education levels of the adult study group are 29% high school not completed, 31% high school completed, 3% business or trade school completed, 21% some college, 12% college graduates, and 4% postbaccalaureate degree [10]. Thus, 55% had completed secondary education and 16% had completed 4 or more yr of college. According to the 1980 Census reports of the general Houston population, 68% have completed secondary education whereas 23.1% have completed 4 or more yr of college [11]. At the 1980 Census, the United States as a whole reported 66.5% of its population, over the age of 25, had 12 or more yr of education while 16.2% had more than 16 yr.

In reviewing the data from the three sample cities (Table 14.1), the San Diego population has a greater proportion of high school graduates than the U.S. average and greater than both Houston and Charlottesville. The Charlottesville area has fewer total high school graduates, but of those who have graduated, many more have completed college than in the other two cities. All three cities have significantly more college graduates than the U.S. average, with Charlottesville being especially remarkable with almost twice as many college graduates as the national average.

These cities were not selected for their census data variance; there are cities with greater diversity that could be selected to demonstrate the great diversity of education level within the communities in the United States. For example, Alaska can boast of 82.5% of its population having at least a high school education and Kentucky only 53.1%. Washington, D.C., reports the

Table 14.1   Years of School Completed, 1980, Percent
of Persons Age 25 yr and over

Location	≥12 yr	≤16 yr
United States	66.5	16.2
Charlottesville	65.1	31
Houston	68.4	23.1
San Diego	78.9	24

U.S. Department of Commerce, Bureau of the Census, *County and City Data Book,* 10th ed., (Washington: U.S. Department of Commerce; 1983).

greatest percentage of individuals with education greater than 16 yr, 27.5%, while West Virginia reports only 10.4%.

MARITAL STATUS

Many authors have written about the effect of traumatic brain injury on the family unit and marital relationship [12,13,14]. Most articles comment on the difficulties of living with a brain-injured person. This research is done on families who remain together, and very few studies comment on the incidence of divorce.

Oddy and Humphrey followed fifty-four patients with severe head injury for 2 yr [15]. Only twelve patients had been married. At 2 yr, only one had divorced, and the authors report that the marriage had been at the point of dissolution at the time of the injury.

In 1972, Walker surveyed the marital status of 146 men who had sustained brain injury during World War II and found that only 11% of them had sought divorce [16]. Also in 1972, Panting and Merry published an article that indicated that 40% of their severely brain-injured subjects were divorced at 2 to 7 yr post injury [17]. In their 1981 article, Mauss-Clum and Ryan reported that one-third of the wives of their sample of thirty brain-injured veterans had considered or filed for divorce [18].

None of these articles mentions the divorce rates for the general population during the time of the assessment. Even if local rates were reported, one could expect that the divorce rate of the brain-injured group might appropriately be higher than the general population since the traumatic brain-injured group tends to be younger.

In the Houston 2 yr study of 1980–1982 [10], the marital status groups are divided into those traumatic brain injuries that are mild, moderate, and severe according to Teasdale and Jennett's description [3]. In the severe group, the divorce rate at 2 yr post injury of those who had been married prior to injury was 5%, 8% were separated, 3% were widowed, and 84% were still

Table 14.2   1980 Divorce Rates (per 1,000 population)

Area	Rate
United States	5.2
Charlottesville	5.2
Houston	8.4
San Diego	5.6

U.S. Department of Commerce, Bureau of the Census, *County and City Data Book,* 10th ed., (Washington: U.S. Department of Commerce; 1983).

married. In the moderate group 12% were divorced, 4% were separated, and 84% were married. In the mild group 1% were divorced, 7% were separated, 4% were widowed, and 87% were married. It is significant to note the divorce rate in Houston during 1980 was 8.4 per 1,000 population [11]. The issue of divorce rates during the study period of the Houston study especially illustrates the need to consider the local norms in the reporting of sociological data at points in time.

The divorce rate in the United States was 5.2 per 1,000 population in 1980. The rate has remained relatively stable since 1979 at 5.3, 5.2 in 1980, 5.3 in 1981, 5.1 in 1982, and 5 in 1983. In 1983 the number of divorces went down for the first time since 1962 [11].

The divorce rate in all the sample cities (Table 14.2) is higher than the national rate, but the Houston rate is 62% greater than the national. One would intuitively expect the divorce rate among traumatically brain-injured individuals to be higher than the local norms because of the severe pressure placed by the residual deficits from the brain injury on the relationship and the average age of the traumatically brain-injured population is younger than the population in general; thus, the marriages would perhaps be more vulnerable. The Houston results did not confirm the intuition. Divorce within the first two years post trauma is not a notable result of incurring traumatic brain injury. This is not to say there are no stresses on the relationships. In addition, the couples may divorce at a point greater than 2 yr post injury. However, at 2 yr the couples were together, and programs to continue to support these couples would appear appropriate.

EMPLOYMENT

The use of return to work as an outcome measure has been criticized by some authors [3]. Although there is merit in these criticisms, perhaps even to the extent that work should not be used as an assessment of outcome, it is significant to know how many traumatically brain-injured individuals eventually re-enter the work force. If one considers the data, not as a measure of outcome but as an indicator of the impact of traumatic brain injury on the community's work force, then most of the criticisms are not applicable.

Comparability of studies on return to work are plagued with problems of defining exactly what is meant by work [19], the assessment of work status at a wide variety of time intervals post injury, the inequality of employment opportunities in the various years(s) in which the studies are done, and the inequality of opportunities in the geographic areas in which the studies are done. Despite the problems, return to work is one of the most prevalent outcome variables discussed in the literature.

In Oddy and Humphrey's head-injured group [15], forty-five of the forty-nine patients seen at 6 mo had been in full-time jobs at the time of injury. Thirty had returned to work within 6 mo after injury, an additional seven by 1 yr, and one more between 1 and 2 yr. Although these authors had a control group, they did not report on the work activity of the control patients. The reader has no idea of the employment potential of a non-head-injured individual at the time of the study.

The study by Dresser et al also employed a control group of veterans who were similar to the head-injured group in age, rank, time of service, and the unit in which they served [6]. In the head-injured group 75% were at work 15 yr after injury while 95% of the controls were working. Although these investigators analyzed the impact of a multitude of factors on the subject's ability to return to work, no mention is made of geographic location of the individuals within each group. No mention is made as to whether the subjects were comparable in rural or urban locations where employment opportunities vary. There is no discussion of individuals who would classify themselves as seeking employment. The basic presumption is that patients who were able to work were working and those who were not working were affected only by their head injury or the 100% disability payments they were receiving.

Gilchrist and Wilkinsen [20] studied a series of eighty-four severely head-injured patients in London from 1963 to 1975. They did a follow-up survey 9 mo to 15 yr after injury on 72% of the patients and found that twenty-eight (39%) were working, seventeen (24%) were in the same job as prior to injury, and eleven (15%) were in different work (usually of a lower grade). Twenty-seven (38%) were at home but not working, all but four of whom were independent in self-care. Thirteen (18%) were in the hospital, four in mental hospitals. Four (6%) had died. It would appear the study was conducted in 1976 and/or 1977. No mention is made as to whether the patients were all from London or various other parts of the country. Since the patients were evaluated at a point from 9 mo to 15 yr after their injury, there is not an equal opportunity for each to have been rehabilitated and achieve employment.

In his article from Ireland, Brennan [21] studied those who had been former inpatients between 1975 to 1977. The work status of 296 head-injured patients was obtained 9 mo following their injury. One hundred thirty were classified as severely injured, of whom 61% had returned to work. Of the 76 moderate and mildly head injured, 88% had returned to work by 9 mo following their injury. The author then discusses other studies of various years and in various countries and cites those that his research confirms or those with which it differs. The reasons he gives for the variances include definition of severe head injury, extent of rehabilitation, and pending litigation. However, he does not address the notion that the employment rates in the geographic areas studied may vary widely. The opportunities to obtain employment and the varying social pressures to do so may be a significant cause for differences. Certainly, to compare employability of the head injured in Ireland, London, and the United States without addressing the geographic and social variances is tenuous.

In a prospective study of central nervous system trauma patients at the University of Virginia Hospital from 1977 through 1979, 424 mildly head-injured patients were identified for follow-up at 3 mo post injury [8]. More than one-third of the patients who had been gainfully employed had not returned to work. Although the authors did not address the issue of the unemployment rate in the Charlottesville community, they did analyze their data with respect to the impact of education, previous employment, and income level. They found these three variables to be better predictors of unemployment than severity of injury, associated injuries, previous head injuries, and health and disability insurance. These results highlight the significance of accounting for sociological parameters in the analysis of outcome results.

In the Houston study [10], patients were contacted at 2 yr post injury in 1982, 1983, and early 1984. Of those who had been employed prior to injury, 90% of the mildly, 80% of the moderately, and 43% of the severely head-injured patients had returned to work. The seventy-six severely head-injured patients who had been working at the time of their injury reported changes in employment status at 2 yr post injury as follows: 20% same job; 3%, same job but having some difficulty at work; 2%, same job title but lighter duties; 7%, promoted; 5%, new job of equal status; 5%, job of lesser status; 52%, unemployed because of injury; 5%, unemployed for reasons other than injury.

The unemployment rate reported for the three sample cities by the Bureau of Labor Statistics for 1982 is shown in Table 14.3. As can be seen, there is considerable difference in unemployment rates for the three cities, with Char-

Table 14.3 1982 Unemployment Rate (per 1,000 population)

Area	Rate
United States	9.7
Charlottesville	4.5
Houston	7
San Diego	9.3

U.S. Department of Commerce, Bureau of the Census, *County and City Data Book*, 10th ed., (Washington: U.S. Department of Commerce; 1983).

Table 14.4 Unemployment Rate in Houston, Texas (per 1,000 population)

Year	Rate
1980	4.2
1981	4.1
1982	7
1983	9.3

lottesville far below the others and the national average. Thus, it could be presumed that any individual seeking employment in these three cities would experience different degrees of ease in finding work based on availability alone.

For the Houston area, however, the single-year data do not present an accurate evaluation of the employment climate at the time. As can be seen in Table 14.4, there was an upward trend in the employment rates. While the oil crisis had hit many parts of the country (forcing the U.S. unemployment average up), Houston did not begin to notice its impact until 1982 and 1983. The city had been booming with people and jobs when it experienced a growth halt that made career opportunities more difficult and layoffs more prominent.

Considering the Houston data in light of these sociological activities further highlights the high rate of employment among the previously employed. It could have been expected that individuals without any injury who were seeking new jobs or trying to retain old jobs were having a degree of difficulty. The fact that these patients had such a high percentage of returning to work was not anticipated.

SUMMARY

After the family and the physician are confident that the traumatically brain-injured patient will survive, new questions arise. What residual deficits will remain, and what impact will they have on the future life of the patient and the family involved? Society, too, asks if it can bear the loss of a fully functioning individual. Complete answers are not provided by an assessment of the probability of physiological and cognitive deficits. Individuals with similar deficits are each capable of developing different methods for coping with or overcoming problems in resuming life's roles. Society has a different view of traumatic brain injury than the individual. Trauma predominantly hits the youth in the community, and if the damage is severe, the youth may not fill any meaningful roles in the community for years. At minimum, the potential of the injured individual to fulfill his roles in the community is altered. At most, others must perform those roles and the structure of the community is altered as a result.

In providing information to physicians, health practitioners, patients, families, legislators, and communities at large, it is important to take time to reflect adequately on the outcome data. Results of research on physiological parameters in the assessment and the management of the traumatically brain injured are more generalizable than research on the resumption of life-style. To allow for accurate interpretation, outcome study results should be tempered by adjusting for sociological variances. These variances can be seen between cities within the United States as well as between the United States and other countries. For example, the education level, divorce rate, and unemployment rate among communities vary. This chapter has illustrated the impact that a few of the sociological variances have on the conclusions and generalization of outcome study results. The sociological variances must be considered when comparing research reports, accounting for change, evaluating patient out-comes, and publishing research.

ACKNOWLEDGMENT

The follow-up research reported from Houston throughout the text was a part of the Central Nervous System Trauma Center and the Comprehensive Central Nervous System Trauma Centers, NINCDS Grants NS14844 and NS92314, whose principal investigator was Philip L. Gildenberg, M.D., Ph.D. The follow-up project results were gained thanks to the meticulous efforts of Kristen Anderson, M.A., and Lou Esposito, B.S., as well as Alex Von Laufen and Trolene Ring, R.N.

REFERENCES

1. Caveness WF. Incidence of craniocerebral trauma in the U.S. in 1976 with trend from 1970 to 1975. Adv Neurol 1979;22:1.
2. Langfitt TW. Measuring the outcome from head injuries. J Neurosurg 1978;48:673–78.
3. Jennett B, Teasdale G. Management of head injuries. Philadelphia: F.A. Davis, 1981.
4. Rosenthal M, Griffith ER, Bond MR, Miller JD. Rehabilitation of the head injured adult. Philadelphia: F.A. Davis, 1983.
5. Becker D, Miller J, Ward J, Greenberg RP, Young HF, Sakalas R. The outcome from severe head injury with early diagnosis and intensive management. J Neurosurg 1977;47:491–502.
6. Dresser M, Meirowsky AM, Weiss GH, McNeel ML, Simon GA, Caveness WF. Gainful employment following head injury. Arch Neurol 1973;29:111–16.
7. Tobis J, Pun K, Sheridan J. Rehabilitation of the severely brain injured patient. Scand J Rehab Med 1982;14:83–88.
8. Jane J, Rimel R, Poberskin L, Tyson G, Steward O, Gennarelli T. Outcome and pathology of head injury. In: Grossman R, Gildenberg P, eds. Head injury: basic and clinical aspects. New York: Raven Press, 1982;229–37.

9. Rimel RW, Giordani B, Barth JT, Jane JA. Moderate head injury: completing the clinical spectrum of brain trauma. Neurosurgery 1982;11:344–51.

10. Wagner K. Brain injury: a prospective outcome study. Paper presented at the fifth annual traumatic head injury conference. Braintree, Mass., October 17–19, 1984.

11. County and city data book, 10th ed. Washington: U.S. Department of Commerce, Bureau of the Census, 1983.

12. Romano MD. Family response to traumatic head injury. Scand J Rehab Med 1974;6:1–4.

13. Rosenbaum M, Najenson T. Changes in life patterns and symptoms of low mood as reported by wives of severely brain injured soldiers. J Consult Clin Psychol 1976;144:881–88.

14. Thomsen IV. The patient with severe head injury and his family. Scand J Rehab Med 1974;6:180–83.

15. Oddy M, Humphrey M. Social recovery during the year following severe head injury. J Neurol Neurosurg Psychol 1980;43:798–802.

16. Walker AE. Long-term evaluation of the social and family adjustment of head injuries. Scand J Rehab Med 1972;4:5–8.

17. Panting P, Merry PH. The long term rehabilitation of severe head injuries with particular reference to the need for social and medical support for the patient's family. J Rehab 1972;38:33–37.

18. Mauss-Clum N, Ryan M. Brain injury and the family. J Neurosurg Nursing 1981;13:165–69.

19. Wagner KA, Brown K, Gildenberg PL, Haar FL, Kaufman HH, Miner ME. Alternative definition of work and their effect on the prediction of outcome in the traumatically brain injured adult. Paper presented at the international symposium on the traumatic brain injured adult and child. Boston, Mass., October 29–31, 1981.

20. Gilchrist E, Wilkinsen M. Some factors determining prognosis in young people with severe head injuries. Arch Neurol 1979;36:355–59.

21. Brennan M. Resumption of work following discharge from hospital. Irish Med J 1981;74:5–7.

Chapter 15

The Current Status of Head Injury Rehabilitation

Karyl M. Hall
D. Nathan Cope

The formal rehabilitation of the traumatically head injured as a distinct clinical entity is a relatively new phenomenon. In 1975 the number of rehabilitation centers with separately identified head injury programs was quite small. Since then, comprehensive rehabilitation of the head-injured patient has undergone accelerated growth, with specifically designed programs now numbering in the hundreds in the United States alone. There has been a concurrent focus by these programs on specific problem areas and approaches, from coma arousal centers through more traditional comprehensive inpatient acute rehabilitation to long-term outpatient transitional and cognitive remediation centers. An increased awareness of the scope of the problem has developed, both at the professional level, indicated by the proliferation of conferences dedicated to this subject, and within the public sector, reflected in the founding and rapid nationwide growth of a consumer advocacy group, the National Head Injury Foundation [1].

These new rehabilitation programs have noted and reflected distinct characteristics and needs of head injury patients. Characteristics include the peak age of incidence (i.e., young adults), the extreme difficulty in making an accurate prognosis, and the typically diffuse rather than focal neurologic lesions. Such diffuse lesions imply both a complexity of neurologic and psychological syndromes and a potentially different course of recovery than that seen in the more localized and dense lesions of stroke. Current clinical opinion seems to recommend early, intense, and long-duration rehabilitation treatment. Such treatment would begin in the neurotrauma intensive care unit (ICU) with coma treatment teams, progress through multidisciplinary acute rehabilitation with the addition of recently developed treatments of cognitive and behavioral deficits, and then to long-term nonhospital transitional or residential-based programs. These programs can extend years post injury.

There has been a lack of rigorous scientific assessment of these new clinical approaches. Particularly difficult has been any attempt to quantify the differential benefit to be obtained by these treatment techniques. This deficiency has a special significance in that many of the reported results of these new approaches, expressed usually in qualitative and clinical rather than quantitative and operational terms, appear to conflict with rather long-held and firmly entrenched ideas concerning neurologic recovery. Traditional concepts consider the brain an organizationally rigid structure with little ability to repair neuronal loss. Recovery that does occur after injury is considered spontaneous and largely independent of environmental influence. Recent rehabilitation approaches consider brain recovery to depend in part on appropriate retraining, taking advantage of the imputed plasticity of the central nervous system (CNS). These opposing viewpoints explain current controversies over what constitutes necessary or optimal clinical treatment.

We want not only to ensure the best clinical outcome but also to assess the cost to obtain this outcome. To state that health care costs are under intense scrutiny is fast becoming banal. Nevertheless, some estimate of cost-effectiveness is a necessary factor in any evaluation of new health care proposals.

Finally, there remains the problem of determining what elements of any particular regimen are effective and which are incidental. Cost-effectiveness evaluation for the treatment of the head injured is a methodologically difficult task, not least due to the interplay of cognitive, behavioral, and social factors in outcome. This is a problem in complexity not unlike that of assessing the value of psychotherapy for mental disturbance, about which research is just now offering scientifically acceptable results in support of definite benefit. Many early studies of psychotherapy failed to show definite advantage, which we now can appreciate as not being equivalent to proving no advantage. It will undoubtedly be equally difficult to demonstrate definitively the benefits of rehabilitation of head injury. Studies in both animals and humans are addressing this issue.

RELEVANT STUDIES

A number of animal studies have renewed interest in the question of CNS plasticity, particularly the question of possible repair of CNS damage. Reviews have dealt with its implications for therapeutic intervention in brain-injured humans [2,3]. It has been pointed out that the injured brain may continue its recovery for years following damage and that sprouting (reactive synaptogenesis) of nearby uninjured axons or unmasking of preexisting but functionally suppressed neural pathways may be the most likely mechanisms involved [4]. Goldman and Lewis pointed out that such recovery in animals is not totally spontaneous [5]. For example, the degree to which monkeys were able to recover performance on a delayed alternation task following orbital prefrontal lesions depended on experience with the task post injury. Such recovery also was contingent to some degree on the temporal proximity of such training to the time of the lesion. Those monkeys whose training was given earlier post lesion tended to have higher recovery scores [6]. Black and co-workers have compared recovery from hemiplegia secondary to motor cortical lesions, and they reported that a more complete ultimate recovery is attained in animals required to use or train the involved limb immediately after injury compared with a matched control group given equivalent training at a later period [7]. Yu concluded in a review of such animal studies that a variety of training paradigms seemed to lead to increased recovery from CNS lesions [8]. Other studies have also shown that direct and active involvement in an enriched or therapeutic environment has a beneficial effect on brain weight, morphology, and chemistry in both normal and brain-lesioned adult animals [9].

There are qualitative as well as quantitative differences between human and animal brain function. Given that these principles of training and recovery may hold in the clinical situation, other problems remain. For example, it appears that in most settings animal recovery is enhanced primarily in the training task and does not generalize to activities outside the test situation. This may imply that such animal results are an interesting but therapeutically irrelevant phenomenon. Caution is needed in applying evidence from animal studies of recovery of function from CNS lesions to the human.

There has been very little rigorous investigation regarding the value of various treatment programs for human traumatic head injury. Rusk and co-workers reviewed 102 head injury patients whose entry into rehabilitation was an average of 20 mo post injury [10]. They reported 30 frozen shoulders, 40 major decubiti, and approximately 200 other major joint deformities. Significant patient gains in health and independence occurred as a result of rehabilitation. In a largely qualitative study, Cogstad and Kjellman reported that functional outcome in a group of head-injured patients was improved when associated with early and continuous rehabilitation [11].

Although there is a paucity of published controlled studies on head injury, evidence regarding the question of benefit of rehabilitation is available for other CNS disabilities. Lehmann et al studied 114 stroke victims admitted to a rehabilitation center and concluded that significant and persistent functional gains were achieved within the rehabilitation stay that could not be attributed simply to spontaneous recovery [12]. Anderson et al found similar results in an evaluation of cerebrovascular accident (CVA) patients [13]. Routine and regular follow-up was needed to maintain gains achieved in rehabilitation. Another study by Anderson and co-workers investigated the difference in mortality and independence in self-care between unmatched groups of rehabilitated and nonrehabilitated CVA patients up to several years post hospitalization [14]. Rehabilitation appeared to have no effect on mortality but had a positive advantage in contributing to quality of life.

Some earlier studies are not as encouraging. Waylonis and Keith compared unmatched groups of patients on functional outcome measures before and after the introduction of a rehabilitation program. They could not demonstrate any impact of the program on outcome [15]. Boyle and Scalzitti studied

478 consecutive CVA admissions and found no relationship between amount of rehabilitation treatment and functional outcome [16]. More seriously involved patients may have received more treatment, which could explain the inability to demonstrate positive findings.

Assuming a benefit to rehabilitation, a closely related issue is the advantage of admission to a rehabilitation unit early after injury as opposed to later. Novack et al reported no functional benefit to CVA patients admitted early to rehabilitation, with the exception of physical therapy measures [17]. However, matched early and late groups were not utilized, leaving the possibility for bias. Smith and Smith, in a randomized, controlled trial of acute stroke patients, found that those rehabilitated early after injury were more often independent in self-care than those rehabilitated later. Findings suggested that early referral rather than the amount or duration of treatment was the critical factor in improved outcome [18]. Other studies also suggest that early institution of rehabilitation leads to greater functional improvement and ultimately superior functional status among CVA patients [19,20].

The analysis of rehabilitation outcome is less complex for spinal cord injury (SCI). The neurologic syndrome is often stable from the time of injury, and functional gains are often an obviously direct result of rehabilitation intervention. Young reported fewer hospital days and substantial savings for early versus late admissions to comprehensive regional SCI centers [21].

One difficulty in interpreting these varied findings lies in the inconsistency of quality of care across centers, with differing treatment philosophies and experience. Results obtained from one center may indeed contradict findings of another, based solely or at least in part on the nature of the treatment provided. For example, Albrecht and Harasymiw compared 230 SCI and focal cerebral patients at ten leading rehabilitation centers [22]. They found that cost-effectiveness varied substantially across centers. An excellent review of the question of cost-effectiveness in CVA and SCI rehabilitation by Johnston and Keith highlights the contradictory findings and the design weaknesses in studies to date [23].

In contrast to the situation in stroke and SCI, there are, other than the study to be reviewed, presently no published reports of a controlled investigation of the benefit due to early comprehensive rehabilitation for traumatic brain injury. The authors, in the course of a 4 yr National Institute of Handicapped Research study on the comprehensive rehabilitation of traumatic head injury, collected descriptive and outcome data sequentially on eighty traumatically brain-injured patients [24]. Subsequent analyses of these data allowed a quasi-experimental treatment and control group comparison between matched patients given early versus late rehabilitation [25].

Specifically, it was hypothesized that patients admitted into an intensive rehabilitation program from acute medical/surgical wards would benefit by a significantly shorter stay in acute rehabilitation and have better functional recovery. Of the eighty patients on whom data had been collected, median days to rehabilitation admission was 35. It happened that all patients admitted within 35 days were in coma fewer than 15 days. This became the early admission group ($n = 16$). Only those patients with coma fewer than 15 days and admission later than 35 days were chosen as the late admission group ($n = 20$). Multiple measures taken at admission were then compared between groups to ensure similarity on potentially biasing factors. No significant differences existed for the admission measures compared (age, length of coma, disability rating, Glasgow Coma Scale, Glasgow Outcome Scale). Five additional measures were compared at 2 mo post injury. Since severity of deficit following brain injury is inversely proportional to time since injury, these 2 mo measures were assessed to compare clinically early and late groups at an equivalent interval post injury. Significant differences were found only for awareness of bowel and bladder function and average psychological impairment, indicating that early rehabilitation admissions were less impaired on these factors. Further comparisons were made of medical and surgical complications in each group. Of six factors, only the number of tracheostomies was significantly greater in the late group. CT scan comparisons yielded no significant differences.

After establishing acceptable comparability between groups, clinical outcome scores and days of acute hospitalization and acute rehabilitation were compared. Table 15.1 shows disability at discharge on the Disability Rating Scale [26] and Glasgow Outcome Scale, as well as on a social status outcome measure rated at 2 yrs post injury for early versus late admissions [24]. It is evident that these outcome scores were not significantly different between groups. Table 15.2 shows the difference in acute care, inpatient rehabilitation, and total hospital days for patients admitted to rehabilitation within 35 days versus greater than 35 days post injury. A dramatic difference of 80 hospital days existed between groups. When this number of hospital days saved is multiplied by a currently conservative $500/day charged for such hospitalization, a reduced cost of $40,000 in hospital charges per patient is estimated for those patients admitted early into comprehensive rehabilitation.

Although this study has some problems, one of which is the small sample size, controlled quasi-experimental studies can provide definitive information on such questions as the effects of rehabilitation on outcome.

DISCUSSION

The theoretical basis for the proposed advantage of early rehabilitation can be argued on two grounds. First, extended total hospitalization may result from a delay or failure to maximize ultimate potential neurologic recovery due to delay in retraining or treatment. There may be a critical period, a therapeutic window, for maximizing recovery by means of rehabilitation, that diminishes with time post injury. Animal studies cited previously support this concept. Second, nonneurologic complications may and often do arise during prolonged residence in an acute medical/surgical unit, which require further treatment and, therefore, increased hospitalization. Rusk's series of patients, cited earlier,

Table 15.1 Comparison of Outcome Measures for Early and Late Rehabilitation Admissions

Instrument	Early Admissions			Late Admissions			t	p
	$\overline{X}$	S.D.	Number	$\overline{X}$	S.D.	Number		
Disability rating at discharge	5.88	2.55	16	5.55	2.63	20	.381	NS
Glasgow outcome scale at discharge	2.94	0.57	16	2.58	0.61	19	1.810	NS
Social status outcome at 2 yr	1.17	1.59	12	2.27	1.79	15	1.689	NS

Reprinted by permission of the Archives of Physical Medicine and Rehabilitation. From Cope DN, Hall K. Head injury rehabilitation: benefit of early intervention. Arch Phys Med Rehabil 1982; 63:433–37.

Table 15.2 Comparison of Length of Hospitalization for Early and Late Rehabilitation Admissions

Variable	Early Admissions			Late Admissions			t	p
	X̄	S.D.	Number	X̄	S.D.	Number		
Acute hospital days	20.9	7	16	55.8	21.9	20	5.940	.001
Acute inpatient rehabilitation days	43.5	36.5	16	88.8	50.3	20	2.634	.01
Total hospital days	64.4	37.2	16	144.6	52.3	20	4.733	.001
Median hospital days	53.5			149				

Reprinted by permission of the Archives of Physical Medicine and Rehabilitation. From Cope DN, Hall K. Head injury rehabilitation: benefit of early intervention. Arch Phys Med Rehabil 1982; 63:433–37.

rehabilitated an average of 20 mo post injury, document a high incidence of such medical complications [10].

In addition, we must not assume that complications of delayed rehabilitation are represented by physical measures of morbidity alone. Multiple studies of long-term outcome have indicated that the most severely disabling features of the head-injured patient are in the psychological or behavioral arena [27,28]. It also appears that these psychological complications are significantly more intense for the head injury patient and his family than for those with other types of severe neurologic disabilities [29]. It is not true that these psychological dysfunctions respond best to simple passage of time or benign neglect. Studies with other types of serious medical conditions have clearly shown the advantages of early and aggressive psychological intervention. For example, in a study of a crisis intervention program in newly diagnosed diabetic children, 223 families were divided into two groups, one which received special crisis intervention counseling at the time of diagnosis and one which received routine education and support. The families that received routine treatment showed significantly greater problems with compliance to the medical program, family relationships, and sociability than the immediately treated group. In addition, the control group subsequently required three times the amount of effort (i.e., time invested in counseling) to bring it to a comparable level of adjustment [30].

It remains for future studies to confirm and extend findings suggesting benefit of early and comprehensive head injury rehabilitation. There is clearly a basic requirement to minimize selection bias on the design of studies. This is ideally accomplished through randomization. However, there are significant ethical issues involved in randomly assigning or restricting treatment that were discussed in Chapter 13. A limited but acceptable alternative would be to match patients within the same center with different treatment characteristics and compare relative outcome. To date this has proven a resistant problem in head injury. The head-injured population clinically has multiple syndromes, and it is difficult for any one center to obtain a reasonably large sample for study.

We currently have limited capability to recognize and measure the prognostic variables most important in outcome. It is essential to do the groundwork of developing comprehensive, sensitive, and reliable instruments to assess outcome. The scale most widely used today, the Glasgow Outcome Scale, has been shown to be too insensitive to assess many rehabilitation aspects of recovery from head injury. Its use may have helped lead to an unnecessarily shortened expectation of length of recovery by many clinicians [26].

The need for a comprehensive outcome scale after brain injury has been recognized, and numerous scales have been published in the literature [31]. A joint committee of the American Academy and the American Congress of Rehabilitation is pursuing development of a reliable set of functional assessment instruments for general use in rehabilitation. Success in this important endeavor should allow comparison of outcome within and across centers [32].

REFERENCES

1. The National Head Injury Foundation. 18A Vernon St. Framingham, MA 01701.
2. Bach-y-Rita P, ed. Recovery of function: theoretical considerations for brain injury rehabilitation. Bern: Hans Huber Publishers and Baltimore: University Park Press, 1980.
3. Finger S, Stein DG. Brain damage and recovery: research and clinical perspectives. New York: Academic Press, 1982.
4. Bach-y-Rita P. Central nervous system lesions: sprouting and unmasking in rehabilitation. Arch Phys Med Rehabil 1981;62:413–17.
5. Goldman PS, Lewis ME. Developmental biology of brain damage and experience. In: Cotman C, ed. Neuronal plasticity. New York: Raven Press, 1978;291–310.
6. Goldman PS. The role of experience in recovery of function following orbital prefrontal lesions in infant monkeys. Neuropsychologia 1976;14:401–12.
7. Black P, Markowitz RS, Cianci SN. Recovery of motor function after lesions in motor cortex of monkeys. In: CIBA Foundation Symposium no. 34. Outcome of severe damage to the central nervous system. Amsterdam: Elsevier, 1975;65–83.
8. Yu J. Functional recovery with and without training following brain damage in experimental animals: a review. Arch Phys Med Rehabil 1976;57:38–41.
9. Rosenzweig MR. Animal models for effects of brain lesions and for rehabilitation. In: Bach-y-Rita P, ed. Recovery of function: theoretical considerations for brain injury rehabilitation. Bern: Hans Huber Publishers, 1980;127–73.
10. Rusk HA, Block JM, Lowman EW. Rehabilitation following traumatic brain damage: Immediate and long-term follow-up results in 127 cases. Med Clin North Am 1969;53:677–84.
11. Cogstad AC, Kjellman AM. Rehabilitation prognosis related to clinical and social factors in brain injured of different etiology. Soc Sci Med 1976;10;283–88.
12. Lehmann JF, DeLateur BJ, Fowler RS, Warren CG, Arnhold R, Schertzer G, Hurka R, Whitmore JJ, Masock AJ, Chambers KH. Stroke: does rehabilitation affect outcome? Arch Phys Med Rehabil 1975;56:375–82.
13. Anderson TP, McClure WJ, Athelstan G, Anderson E, Crewe N, Arndts L, Ferguson MB, Baldridge M, Gullickson G Jr, Kottke FJ. Stroke rehabilitation: evaluation of its quality by assessing patient outcomes. Arch Phys Med Rehabil 1978;59:170–75.
14. Anderson TP, Baldridge M, Ettinger MG. Quality of care for completed stroke without rehabilitation: evaluation by assessing patient outcomes. Arch Phys Med Rehabil 1979;60:103–07.
15. Waylonis GW, Keith MW. Stroke rehabilitation in midwestern county. Arch Phys Med Rehabil 1973;54:151–55.
16. Boyle RW, Scalzitti PD. Study of 480 consecutive cases of cerebral vascular accident. Arch Phys Med Rehabil 1963;44:19–28.
17. Novack TA, Satterfield WT, Lyons K, Kolski G, Hackmeyer L, Connor M. Stroke onset and rehabilitation: time lag as a factor in treatment outcome. Arch Phys Med Rehabil 1984;65:316–19.
18. Smith ME, Smith DL. Therapy impact on functional outcome in a controlled trial of stroke rehabilitation. Arch Phys Med Rehabil 1982;63:21–24.
19. Feigenson JS. Stroke rehabilitation: effectiveness, benefits and costs. Some practical considerations. Stroke 1979;10:1–4.

20. Truscott BL, Kretschmann CM, Toole JF, Pajak TF. Early rehabilitative care in community hospitals: effects on quality of survivorship following stroke. Stroke 1974;5:623–29.
21. Young JS. Hospital study report. Model Systems' SCI Digest 1979;1:11–32.
22. Albrecht GL, Harasymiw SJ. Evaluating rehabilitation outcome by cost function indicators. J Chron Dis 1979;32:525–33.
23. Johnston MV, Keith RA. Cost-benefits of medical rehabilitation: review and critique. Arch Phys Med Rehabil 1983;64:147–54.
24. Head Injury Rehabilitation Project. Final Report: Severe head trauma—comprehensive medical approach (collaborative). Project 13-P-59156/9. San Jose: Institute for Medical Research at Santa Clara Valley Medical Center, 1982.
25. Cope DN, Hall K. Head injury rehabilitation: benefit of early intervention. Arch Phys Med Rehabil 1982;63:433–37.
26. Hall K, Cope DN, Rappaport MR. Glasgow Outcome Scale and Disability Rating Scale: comparative usefulness in following recovery in traumatic head injury. Arch Phys Med Rehabil 1985;66:35–37.
27. Brooks DN, McKinlay W. Personality and behavioural change after severe blunt head injury—a relative's view. J Neurolog Neurosurg and Psychiatry 1983;46:336–44.
28. Bond MR, Brooks DN, McKinlay W. Burdens imposed on the relatives of those with severe brain damage due to injury. Acta Neurochir (Suppl.) (Wien) 1979;28:124–25.
29. Rosenbaum M, Najenson T. Changes in life patterns and symptoms of low mood as reported by wives of severely brain-injured soldiers. J Consult Clin Psychol 1976;44:881–88.
30. Galatzer A, Amir S, Gil R, Karp M, Laron Z. Crisis intervention program in newly diabetic children. Diabetes Care 1982;5:414–19.
31. Forer S. Functional assessment instruments in medical rehabilitation. J Organization of Rehab Evaluators 1982;2:29–41.
32. American Congress of Rehabilitation Medicine/American Academy of Physical Medicine and Rehabilitation Task Force. Uniform National Data System. For further information, contact Steven Forer, Rehabilitation Services Manager, Santa Clara Valley Medical Center, 751 So. Bascom Avenue, San Jose, CA 95128.

Chapter 16

Recovery versus Outcome after Head Injury in Children

Michael E. Miner
Jack M. Fletcher
Linda Ewing-Cobbs

Head injury is a major cause of death in children, yet neurosurgeons treating severely head-injured children report extremely good results in those children who survive [1,2,3]. The determination of the quality of survival has enormous impact on the patients and their families, but this is true of all disorders of children. Since pediatric head injuries account for up to one out of every six hospital admissions in children, the question of outcome has great impact on allotment of acute care medical resources [4]. These cases are extremely expensive in terms of medical care dollars and personnel time. However, if outcome is outstanding then every effort should be made to salvage the life of any child regardless of the severity of brain injury.

When discussing such cases with neurosurgeons and after reviewing the neurosurgery literature, one might easily come to the conclusion that survival guarantees a good outcome after brain injury in children. However, the quality of survival of head-injured children has been increasingly scrutinized, and serious doubt has been brought to bear on the good results reported in the neurosurgery literature. This scrutinizing is important because if outcome is not as perfect as previously reported, a closer look at rehabilitation efforts and education for these children may be required. We have been in a unique position to compare the results described by a neurosurgeon who treats and follows a large number of head-injured children to the results obtained by neuropsychologists examining the same patients.

METHODS OF OUTCOME EVALUATION

Evaluating children after head injury is a difficult problem. One desires enough information not only to categorize the patients for comparative purposes but also to have an impact on rehabilitative efforts. Rapidity of evaluation is of no

233

small import to the busy clinician, but a detailed assessment is also required for definitive evaluation. Methods of determining global outcome are numerous, but they are generally vague and imprecise.

Glasgow Outcome Scale

One tool utilized in evaluating both children and adults is the Glasgow Outcome Scale [5]. The utility of this method of outcome assessment is that it is simple, quickly performed, and anyone, including neurosurgeons, can use it. It is a five category scale, ranging from good recovery to death.

Good Recovery

A good recovery allows for some persistent sequelae, but the patient is capable of returning to work; in children, work is equated with school. Therefore, one of the major criteria for determining a good outcome in a child is the ability to return to school. In the preschool child such a clear-cut definition of work is not readily available, but common sense allows an evaluator to make a reasonable assessment.

Moderate Disability

The key terms in this category are *independence* and *disability*. Independence has vague meaning in assessing disability in children because by definition they are dependent. Even more difficult is the concept of self-care in children because of its vagueness and sociologic implications. Fortunately, common sense once again comes to the rescue. One simply deletes these as criteria in the child less than 5 yr of age and depends on the presence of specific deficits to assess the degree of disability.

Severe Disability

A conscious child who has a dependent existence is clearly severely disabled. There may be some difficulty in determining the precise severity of disability, especially in infants, but rarely are these patients difficult to identify. Such children may be candidates for institutionalization.

Vegetative

Nonsentient survival requires minimal sophistication to identify.

Death

By definition, this is the most clearly defined category and the category indicating the poorest outcome.

The major concern with the application of the Glasgow Outcome Scale in children is primarily between the good recovery and the moderate disability categories. The remaining categories are much easier to define and appear to occur infrequently.

Karnofsky Scale

The Karnofsky Scale is a work-related scale that has been used to record the status of a variety of patient groups. Definitions of adult work are not always easily transcribed to the child, but the assessment is not difficult and represents a widely used outcome scoring system. A score of 80 or greater implies that the patient requires no special care. A score of 50 is associated with near institutionalization status. Assessment by both the Glasgow Outcome Scale and the Karnofsky Scale are rapidly performed, and the interobserver differences are small.

Neuropsychological Evaluation

In contrast to the neurosurgeon's methods of evaluating outcome, the neuropsychologist's evaluation is time consuming and detailed. In these evaluations, patients are tested for 2 to 3 hr, but each test is scored at a later time, resulting in the patient's receiving a relatively delayed determination of status. Memory, attention, constructional and language skills, and academic achievement and somatosensory function are recorded in detail [6]. To compare outcomes with the neurosurgeon's evaluation, the neuropsychological results were placed in four categories.

An evaluation of *excellent* meant that the child was within one standard deviation of the norm in each tested category. Excellent did not necessarily mean no deficits from the parents' viewpoint but rather no differences from the average child of the same age. This score does not mean that the child was recovered to an average level but that the child is not clearly abnormal. A patient with a *mild* disability was deficient in one or two neuropsychological categories, and a patient with a *moderate* disability was deficient in three or four. The *mentally deficient* category applied to those patients who were more than one standard deviation away from average normative standards in all categories.

Correlation between the neuropsychologist's mentally deficient category and the Glasgow Outcome Scale's severe disability and vegetative survival are clear. Good recovery and moderate disability are less obviously correlated with the neuropsychological evaluations of excellent, mild, and moderate deficits. However, if the outcome from severe head injury in children is good, then one would expect those with a Glasgow Outcome Scale of good recovery to have an excellent neuropsychological outcome and those with a moderate disability to have mild or moderate cognitive deficits.

PATIENT POPULATION

Twenty patients with moderate to severe head injuries, whose mean age was 5.1 yr, were aggressively treated and followed carefully as outpatients. All modalities of treatment within our resources were utilized while they were in the hospital and as outpatients. They were evaluated at 3 mo intervals for 1 yr following their injury. All outcome evaluations were based on the 1 yr postinjury follow-up.

At the time of hospital admission, the best response in three of the patients was pathologic posturing to deep pain with no response to voice, touch, or mildly painful stimuli. Sixteen would be classified in the severely injured category in terms of their initial neurologic status; that is, a Glasgow Outcome Scale score of 8 or less. Their brain pathology, as evidenced by their initial computerized tomographic (CT) brain scan, was striking in that sixteen of the twenty had major lesions and the other four had less striking CT scans but still were clearly abnormal. Nine of the twenty had early surgical procedures for removal of devitalized brain or hematomas. All but two required mechanical ventilation for some period of time after their injury. It is interesting to note that one-third of these children improved, one-third were unchanged, and one-third worsened within the first 24 hr after injury. Many were in the hospital for prolonged periods of time, and all required some form of outpatient therapy after leaving the hospital. Several required extensive multimodality therapy. Thus, all were sick but not moribund. Most would have been expected to survive, however.

DISCUSSION

Table 16.1 presents the results of the various outcome assessments—the Glasgow Coma Scale scores on admission and at 24 hr and the pathologic diagnosis—for these twenty children. Considering the severity of their injuries, all but two patients had recovered well by 1 yr after injury according to the neurosurgical evaluator. Both their Glasgow Outcome Scale scores and their ratings on the Karnofsky Scale were exciting. The remaining two patients were clearly devastated. Thus, the children fell into one of two categories of outcome—good or severe. These findings are in agreement with those of other investigators and give credence to the notion that children usually do well after severe head injuries.

It is interesting that the outcomes defined by neuropsychological testing are also not surprising when compared with information available in the neuropsychology literature [7–12]. There was a continuum of outcome by neuropsychological testing rather than two categories as observed by the neurosurgeon. Most important, however, is the magnitude of the difference in outcome assessment between the neurosurgical and neuropsychological evaluation. All but one of the eighteen children with good outcomes had major difficulties 1

Table 16.1 Results of Outcome Assessments

| Age | Glasgow Coma Scale Score | | CT Diagnosis | Outcome at 1 yr | | |
	At Admission	After 24 hr		Glasgow Outcome Scale	Karnofsky Scale	Neuropsychology Evaluation
10 yr	4	6	Basal ganglion hematoma	Good	100	Mild
4 yr	5	4	Basal ganglion hematoma	Severe	50	Severe
2 yr	6	6	GSW left hemisphere	Good	80	Moderate
1 yr	6	6	Subdural hematoma hemisphere infarct	Severe	50	Severe
6 yr	6	3	Multilobar intracerebral hematoma	Good	90	Moderate
15 yr	6	6	Frontal contusion	Good	100	Mild
13 yr	6	6	Frontal-parietal contusion	Good	100	Moderate
6 yr	7	6	Depressed skull fracture	Good	100	Mild
2 yr	7	7	Diffuse injury	Good	90	Moderate
2 yr	7	7	Parietal hemorrhage	Good	90	Moderate
4 yr	8	7	Midbrain contusion	Good	90	Moderate
8 yr	8	11	Epidural hematoma	Good	100	Mild
2 yr	8	6	Temporal contusion	Good	90	Moderate
1 yr	8	6	GSW right hemisphere	Good	90	Moderate
4 yr	8	14	Diffuse injury	Good	90	Mild
4 yr	9	10	GSW left hemisphere	Good	100	Mild
9 yr	9	10	Diffuse injury	Good	90	Mild
2 yr	10	10	Subdural hematoma	Good	100	Mild
3 mo	10	14	Subdural hematoma	Good	100	Excellent
7 yr	11	11	GSW-temporal acute hydrocephalus	Good	100	Mild

yr after their injury. All eighteen were clearly much recovered from their initial evaluation, but only one conforms to the neuropsychological notion of an excellent outcome. Of these eighteen children, only this child was not receiving special education at 1 yr post injury.

The problem with the information on the outcome of these patients is not that the expectations of either group of observers were violated but that the same patients were being evaluated by two different groups of observers utilizing two significantly different methods. The results are greatly at odds, and we must discover which approach was correct because many major decisions that affect these children depend on the assessment of their status.

The dilemma stems from the diversity of testing methods and the purposes for which the resultant data will be utilized. The importance of evaluating the data can hardly be overemphasized, not only for the purpose of patient care decisions but also for many broader issues such as allocation of medical resources, use of child restraints in automobiles, funding of projects for the handicapped, early childhood development projects, and many others. Only by carefully describing the results of current therapy for any disease can we establish the need for a new treatment program.

There are several methods by which outcome after head injury can be described, each with merit. The most obvious method, and the most fundamental, is survival statistics. Such data have great value in demographic studies and to emergency medical personnel, but the limitations are obvious.

Similarly, evaluation of traditional neurologic function is important, but it may have little relationship to how the patient functions physically, emotionally, or socially and may be a poor guide to long-term therapy. This is especially true in children who seem to do particularly well by the classic neurologic examination but rather poorly when their higher cognitive skills are evaluated. Unfortunately, traditional signs of neurologic deficit show rapid recovery after head injury, but higher cortical function often remains impaired [10].

Evaluation of the functional status is extremely helpful in defining recovery and therapy regimens. However, functional status evaluations like the Karnofsky Scale may fail to depict outcome accurately in the sense of integration into the patient's previous milieu. The recognition of this difficulty has spurred efforts to evaluate higher cortical function. We ultimately want to know how injured children are able to learn, integrate into peer groups, and be in control of their behavior. We have experiential reasons to believe that these factors will be more predictive of long-term recovery after head injury than any of the foregoing. In addition, only through this type of understanding can educationally interactive regimens be evaluated; that is, if we are interested in how a child is learning, we must devise testing schemes that incorporate tests of the substrate for learning.

The next level of testing could be in terms of behavior. Persons experienced in treating head-injured children recognize that there are changes in behavior in many of these children, but few data are available on this topic.

Rutler has shown that patients with severe head injuries frequently have significant changes in behavior [13]. These studies imply that behavioral adjustment may well be the most important influence on those patients who have excellent outcomes but are not back to normal.

However, as research progresses, we may well find that outcome testing should be based on a hierarchy. As one level of testing identifies recovery of function, the child continues to the next level of evaluation. First must come survival and recovery of motor and primary sensory function. Certainly hemiparetic, blind, or deaf children can learn and become independent, but we do expect that their physical disability will affect their function. Such recovery scoring may appropriately guide the child's total therapy program. Functional scales of recovery are also useful guides to therapeutic decisions—e.g., when it is appropriate for the family to take over the day-to-day care of their child. Similarly, they can guide the therapist in adding and deleting treatment regimens. However, scales can define recovery but not the essence of outcome.

The essence of outcome is extremely difficult to measure and must always be couched with significant disclaimers. We must acknowledge that we do not know when children cease to recover after brain injury. One must also recognize that a good outcome is in the eyes of the observer. However, the important view is that of the child's recovery, physically, psychologically, intellectually, and emotionally. To decide that outcome is good or bad on the basis of one level of testing is to do a disservice to the child.

The issue of the child as a developing organism must also be taken into account. We would not grade highly the 2 yr outcome of a child injured at age 2 yr, who at the age of 4 functioned as a 2-yr-old, even though the child had attained his premorbid level of function. Some of the rules are different for children than for adults. Outcome in children must account for time in terms of expected maturation, usually an insignificant parameter in adults.

SUMMARY

As a group these children had severe injuries with major pathological brain lesions. They were treated by an aggressive regimen with long-term rehabilitative efforts. Their follow-up evaluation illustrates the importance of choosing an outcome scale appropriate to the patient's needs. If these children are judged as having a good outcome as indicated by the Glasgow Outcome and Karnofsky Scales, then no therapeutic interventions are needed. If outcome means that memory, attention, and language skills should be investigated, then the global outcome scores may not have great utility. Furthermore, if the global categories are used by those who do not understand their significance, grievous errors may be made because a good result requires no further treatment. If that assumption is made from the good result category of the Glasgow Outcome Scale, it is in error. We found that the neuropsychological evaluation provided a much more realistic picture of the child's level of functioning. It may be true that the neuropsychologist's evaluation of excellent is also not all the word implies. As we increase our sophistication in evaluating, we may also increase our sophistication in treatment. A hierarchy of evaluation has great appeal with regard to efficiency and appropriate use of personnel. One of our current goals is to suggest when to evaluate each set of parameters so that the evaluation regimen continues to have an impact on rehabilitation and unnecessary treatments are avoided.

REFERENCES

1. Brink JD, Imbus C, Woo-Sam J. Physical recovery after severe closed head trauma in children and adolescents. J Peds 1980;97:721–27.
2. Bruce DA, Schut L, Bruno LA, Woods JH, Sutton LN. Outcome following severe head injury in children. J Neurosurg 1978;48:679–88.
3. Hendrick EB, Harwood-Nash DCF, Hudson AR. Head injuries in children: a survey of 4465 consecutive cases at the Hospital for Sick Children, Toronto, Canada. Clin Neurosurg 1964;11:46–59.
4. Field JH. Epidemiology of head injury in England and Wales with particular application to rehabilitation. Leicester: Printed for HM Stationery Office by Willsons, 1976.
5. Jennett B, Bond M. Assessment of outcome after severe brain damage. Lancet 1975;1:480–87.
6. Tayler HG, Fletcher JM, Satz P. Neuropsychological evaluation of children. In: Goldstein G, Hersen M, eds. Handbook of psychological assessment. New York: Pergamon, 1984;211–34.
7. Flach J, Malmros R. A long-term follow-up study of children with severe head injury. Scand J Rehab Med 1972;4:9–15.
8. Fletcher JM, Ewing-Cobbs L, McLaughlin EJ, Levin HS. Cognitive and psychological sequelae of head injury. In: Brooks BF, Hoelzer DJ, eds. The injured child. Austin: University of Texas Press, 1985;30–39.
9. Levin HS, Eisenberg HM. Neuropsychological impairment after closed head injury in children and adolescents. J Ped Psych 1979;4:389–402.
10. Levin HS, Eisenberg HM, Miner ME. Neuropsychological findings in head injured children. In: Shapiro K, ed. Pediatric head trauma. New York: Futura Publishing Co., 1983;223–40.
11. Mahoney WJ, D'Souza BJ, Haller JA, Rogers MC, Epstein MH, Freeman JM. Long-term outcome of children with severe head trauma and prolonged coma. Pediatrics 1983;5:471–82.
12. Richardson F. Some effects of severe head injury: a follow-up study of children and adolescents after protracted coma. Dev Med Child Neurol 1963;5:471–82.
13. Rutler M. Developmental neuropsychiatry: concepts, issues and problems. J Clin Neuropsych 1982;4:91–115.

Chapter 17

Injury Prevention
Stanley F. Handel
Daniel P. Perales

If the United States were at war and sustaining 150,000 fatalities and millions of other casualties yearly with no end in sight, there is little doubt that national outrage would terminate involvement in that war. Those numbers are tragically real and represent casualties occurring in the United States as a result of intentional and unintentional injuries [1,2].

That our society has not been able to diminish this carnage effectively represents an ongoing national scandal. Possible reasons for this failure include the diffuse multicausal basis of injuries, awareness of injury as a problem being diminished by sporadic occurrence, attitudes that view injury as an act of God or as randomly occurring accidents that cannot be avoided, and a cultural acceptance of violence. Moreover, the economic implications of death and disability resulting from injury have not been widely understood. For these reasons we believe that the individual and societal consequences of injury have been accepted virtually as a built-in cost of our society's activities. These perspectives have blunted any strong public consensus that, on moral grounds alone, a just and humane society must not allow such an epidemic to continue. The issues are fourfold: public health, moral, social, and economic.

SCOPE OF THE PROBLEM

A few statistics illustrate the magnitude of the injury problem in the United States. The approximately 150,000 deaths annually in the United States from injuries result in a death rate of about 1 per 2,000. Traffic deaths alone are in excess of 42,000 per year [3]. Firearm deaths are second only to motor vehicle deaths as a cause of fatal injury and in 1980 accounted for nearly 34,000 fatalities [4]. For all ages, injuries are the fourth leading cause of death after heart disease, cancer, and cerebrovascular disease [5]. In the United States, for people ages 1 through 44, injuries are the leading cause of death. From another viewpoint, if we look at the preretirement years of life lost from

241

intentional and unintentional causes, injuries are the primary cause of years of productive life lost in the United States.

Young males in particular bear the brunt of fatal and serious injury from nearly all causes. At current rates, it is estimated that 1 in every 120 males reaching age 15 will be dead from traffic injuries before age 25. One in every 410 males reaching age 15 will die by homicide before age 25, primarily from firearms. Overall, motor vehicle injuries, other unintentional injuries, homicide, and suicide will claim one in 60 males between their fifteenth and twenty-fifth birthdays [6].

Brain injury due to trauma is a problem of great social and economic importance. Traffic crashes alone account for nearly 180,000 of the estimated 410,000 new cases of brain injury sustained annually in the United States [7]. Males, especially those aged between 15 and 25 yr, account for almost 70% of brain injuries caused by motor vehicle crashes [8]. Although females lag far behind males in the injury statistics, mortality and morbidity from trauma are still substantial problems for them. This has become more apparent as we increasingly recognize rape and wife, child, and parental abuse as crimes of violence.

Examining statistics is useful and allows us to be dispassionate. Nearly all of us, however, have had some degree of personal involvement with severe injury or its possibility. For example, while driving along the freeway a car suddenly careens past on your side of the freeway going in the opposite direction. This can happen very fast, leaving you greatly shaken yet feeling fortunate. Some people are not as lucky. A young research scientist, on his way home after working late at the Department of Neurosurgery at the University of Texas Medical School in Houston, was killed when struck head on by a drunken driver who was driving on the wrong side of the road. In such instances the statistics are meaningless. The sense of personal loss, outrage, and the immorality of the tragedy are overwhelming.

Most of us can probably assemble a list of friends, acquaintances, students, and young professionals who died from traffic trauma, other unintentional injuries, murder, and suicide—an appallingly long list of young, healthy, productive lives brutally terminated. These are no longer statistics but personal affronts. As a society we must realize the need for a major investment in protecting ourselves through the development and implementation of injury prevention. At the individual cognitive level, we must accept that unless motivated to action, we, our families, and friends face more of the same in society's terrible, undeclared war on itself.

COSTS OF INJURY

An American Trauma Society position paper places direct expenses and indirect losses from nonintentional injury at around $63 billion annually and estimates these costs to reach $100 billion by 1985 [2]. Hartunian and co-workers have reported that direct and indirect costs of motor vehicle injuries alone are surpassed only by those incurred by cancer [9]. Overall, injuries may represent the most costly health problem in the United States. As an example of the onus that nonfatal injuries place on society's health resources, of the top three causes of visits to physicians and other contacts for treatment, injuries ranked before heart and respiratory diseases [10]. However, trauma has other costs that are not monetary and include pain, suffering, anger, fear, guilt, and reduced intellect—the human potential never achieved.

One incalculable cost is the negative effect of such an immense diversion of resources from research on cancer, cardiovascular and other diseases, and social intervention efforts. Even though society has been seemingly willing and able to bear the expense, we will never know the opportunities lost if this money had been channeled elsewhere or what contributions those millions of fatalities over the years would have made to our society and culture.

As bleak as these statistics seem, there is hope, as evidenced by downward movement in some statistics—notably, traffic fatalities, which have fallen from a high of 55,000 in 1972 to about 43,000 in 1983 [11]. The decline has not been progressive. Factors cited include the 55 mph speed limit and the economic recession. Complacency must be avoided because the statistics may again rise dramatically. Even if they do not rise, the welcomed decrease in automobile fatalities leaves much to be desired.

ALCOHOL AND DRUGS

Substance abuse is a common thread in the problem of intentional and unintentional injuries. However, alcohol abuse is predominant as the biggest single behavioral manifestation underlying injuries, whether they are traffic crashes, domestic violence, homicides, or suicides [5,12,13]. As many as half the motor vehicle crashes may involve alcohol. There is new evidence that drinking may be involved in as many as 80 to 90% of motor vehicle crashes involving fatalities [3]. It is also noteworthy that crashes in which alcohol plays a role tend to be worse than others. On weekend nights, as many as 10% of all drivers have blood-alcohol content levels that exceed statutory limits.

INJURY AS A PREVENTABLE PUBLIC HEALTH PROBLEM

Society must free itself of the concept that accidents are inevitable. This concept must be replaced with the understanding that many serious injuries and fatalities are preventable. Our society must learn that injuries can be reduced meaningfully by proven intervention methodologies and that epidemiologic research, as in other disease processes, can lead to real advances.

Dr. William Haddon, deceased president of the Insurance Institute for Highway Safety, was one of the world's leading proponents of viewing injury epidemiologically [14]. He and others showed that injuries have point epidemics, seasonal variation, and long-term trends in addition to geographic, socioeconomic, and urban-rural distributions, just as other traditionally recognized disease processes.

Haddon identified energy as the agent of disease with injury resulting from the transfer of larger amounts of energy to the host than the organism can handle without cellular or subcellular harmful effects [14]. The energy may be mechanical, thermal, chemical, or radiant. The agent is transferred to the host by a living organism (a vector) or an inanimate object (a vehicle), with modification superimposed by the environment. The epidemiologists have summarized this concept in terms that medical and public health workers can understand, and just as with other disease processes, rational intercept points for prevention can be identified. Haddon proposed a matrix to help identify those intercept points. The matrix divides damaging interactions into three natural stages: (1) pre-event, (2) event, and (3) postevent, and looks at three factors: (1) human, (2) vehicle (or vector), and (3) environment (or physical and sociocultural) at each stage. This matrix provides the means for identifying prior and possible resource allocations and activities in addition to the efficacies of each, the relevant research and knowledge available and needed, and the priorities for countermeasures judged in terms of cost and decreases in the problem.

Another important contribution by Dr. Haddon to the epidemiologic study of injury was his ten strategies for reducing damage from the various forms that energy takes [14]. The strategies may be summarized as follows:

1. Prevent creation of a hazard.
2. Reduce the amount of hazard brought into being.
3. Prevent the release of the hazard already existing.
4. Modify the rate of spatial distribution of the release of hazard from its source.
5. Separate in time or space the hazard and that to be protected.
6. Separate hazard and that to be protected by a material barrier.
7. Modify basic qualities of the hazard.
8. Make that which is to be protected more resistant to damage from the hazard.
9. Begin to counter the damage already being done by the environmental hazard.
10. Stabilize, repair, and rehabilitate the object of the damage.

Two important points about the ten strategies for injury prevention should be noted. First, Haddon's approaches provide a format for considering and proposing actions for specific injury prevention problems, each of which must be dealt with appropriately. Second, the analysis does not center on causation but on reducing morbidity and mortality.

ACTIVE VERSUS PASSIVE PREVENTION STRATEGIES

When major public health disease prevention methods are examined, it is clear that efforts are most successful when applied in a comprehensive fashion and at proper intersection or intervention points—e.g., having all children immunized through cooperation of schools, legal authorities, physicians, and the public health apparatus. Individual compliance is mandatory and the network is such that compliance is virtually assured. Furthermore, only several well-defined personal actions are necessary over the lifetime. Another example, central purification of drinking water systems, protects the population without need for individual action. Public health measures tend to be least successful when they are dependent on repeated individual behavior and action. How successful would water purification be if the system relied on individuals' purifying their own water supplies? Preventing hazards related to tobacco use has been frustrating because the main strategy has been to influence individual action by modifying behavior. Similarly, in the United States seat belt use efforts have failed. Despite repeated public education campaigns, some of which have been intense and well monitored, relatively little gain has been achieved in terms of the number of people wearing seat belts. Currently, use is in the range of 10 to 20% of the driving public [15]. Federal regulations will require passive restraint systems in motor vehicles if a sufficient number of states do not pass mandatory seat belt use laws. The ultimate effectiveness of this change in seat belt use strategy remains to be seen.

To illustrate the active (or individual action) versus passive (or automatic) strategies, the seat belt example can be used. The automobile industry and others favoring the active strategy place the responsibility on the individual to buckle up, whereas proponents of automatic (passive) measures urge strategies such as automatic seat belts or air bags that do not require the need for repeated individual actions. We are convinced that the injury problem in the United States is so great that an emphasis on automatic, or passive, measures is necessary to achieve reduction of injury morbidity and mortality in general and from the automobile specifically. That is not to say that individual incentives and behavior modifications should not be pursued, but it seems unlikely that a suitable decrease in mortality and morbidity would occur from such efforts. When considering everyday life, acceptance of automatic safety devices is widespread. No one would propose that drivers manually switch on rear lights when braking nor would most people argue the importance of the passive protection provided by smoke alarms and sprinkler systems. The crux of an automatic system's use for injury prevention may be cost and public perception of its relevance. We believe that society really cannot afford to lack well-conceived intervention programs in view of the staggering direct and indirect costs of injury. Lack of action is caused by entrenched beliefs and biases and failure to grasp the economic and moral implications of injury.

SOLUTIONS

Increased national awareness of the injury problem's magnitude is crucial. We must acknowledge injury as a moral issue that is also important socially and economically and that, through the proper application of well-demonstrated strategies, the size of the problem can be diminished. Private sector and public leaders, the public health and medical communities, and the education system must demand safety as an integral part of everyday life. For example, in terms of the largest injury producer in the United States, the automobile, we must demand vehicles that are constructed with safety as a foremost consideration. If there is sufficient compressible space in the periphery of the automobile without impinging on the passenger compartment, if the passenger is appropriately restrained with automatic systems, if the interior of the automobile is properly designed without hard or sharp protuberances, if there is ample room for head deceleration without impact, and if speed is better controlled, then the injury and mortality rate from auto crashes would drop significantly. In tandem, well-designed highways and programs to cope with alcohol and drug problems would further reduce the human highway toll [11].

Research

Research into all aspects of injury prevention, including safety engineering, behavior modification, and other countermeasures, is needed. An accurate injury data base is essential [16,17]. The data base is currently incomplete and faulty, although a properly attained sampling of as little as 2% of injuries could be valid [16]. Much of the current data come from law enforcement sources that collect data primarily for purposes of showing fault and documenting the basis for criminal charges. The information obtained is not the type needed for epidemiology and prevention. National, state, and regional injury registries are needed to define the problem fully and to provide a factual basis for prevention strategies. Virginia became the first state to require reporting of brain injury with the inception of their brain injury registry [7].

Much remains to be done with the issue of driving while under the influence of alcohol and other drugs [18]. The Presidential Commission on Drunk Driving has made the following recommendations:

Uniform age of 21 for alcohol purchase (this is based on the premise that raising the legal age of alcohol purchase to 21 results in a decrease in morbidity and mortality for 18-to-20-yr-olds. It is possible that studies would show that injury from other causes also decreases for this age group.);

Administrative license suspension for blood alcohol levels of 0.1% or more;

Having a 0.08% blood alcohol level as evidence of driving under the influence of alcohol;

Having a 0.1% level as illegal per se;

Substantial fines with no judicial discretion for first-time offenders;

For first violation:
  License suspended 90 day or more,
  100 hr community service, or
  48 hr in jail;

Stiffer penalties for repeaters;

Dramshop laws;

Open container laws

Uniform traffic system and one license-one record for drivers;

Child restraint and safety belt use laws;

Selective enforcement methods and roadblocks to screen for drunken drivers.

Of some note is that this presidential commission did not call for passive countermeasures involving the automobile. However, all drivers, including drunk drivers, should be protected by such measures.

Role of Physicians and Other Health Practitioners

Health practitioners must understand the basic concepts of injury and injury prevention as they understand other disease processes. They must incorporate these sound principles into personal living and health practices to influence families, friends, and patients. Recall the favorable publicity about the influence on the public of physicians who quit smoking. A similar poll is needed of physicians who use seat belts.

Health practitioners can acquire and disseminate information about injury prevention in a variety of ways. They and their assistants can focus on the individual patient and the patient's family with counseling and advice based on factual data. For example, the health practitioner can incorporate recommendations on safe automobiles into patient counseling. A substantial dent in sales of certain models might lead to the automotive industry's finally accepting the concept that the public considers safety important. We might see the elimination of certain models of small cars that have nearly three times the overall injury rate of many full-size station wagons. Information on the relative safety of various automobile models is available through the Insurance Institute for Highway Safety [19]. This is well-researched information that health practitioners can pass on to their patients.

In effect, physicians and other health professionals can be injury prevention activists in their communities. At least some small percentage of professional medical activity and the activities of professional medical organizations should be devoted to injury prevention. This should be especially true for physicians and societies dealing with trauma. The American Academy of Pediatrics is an example of an organization that is increasingly involved with injury prevention.

The Houston-Galveston Injury Prevention Group

Approximately 3 yr ago, a group of concerned men and women, representing a number of disciplines including family practice, public health, neurosurgery, pathology, psychiatry, and radiology, realized the importance of local injury prevention efforts and organized an informal injury prevention group. The group was concerned specifically with the severity of the problem and the scanty resources directed at prevention. After securing a grant from the Moody Foundation of Galveston, the group presented a conference in May 1982 that brought together national, state, and local leaders working in or concerned with injury prevention. This conference issued a formal report, which was presented to the governor and legislature of Texas, highlighting problems of intentional and unintentional injuries in Texas [20]. Through the conference and the report, the Houston-Galveston Injury Prevention Group (H/G-IPG) was able to have some stimulatory and complementary effect on increased injury prevention activities in Texas.

Cooperation and networking has extended to the Texas Medical Association, the Texas Department of Health, and a pediatric child safety restraint coalition. The H/G-IPG testified before the Texas Legislative Subcommittee on Health Care Cost Containment in 1984 about injury prevention as a means of health care cost containment. The testimony, describing the possible cost savings from the implementation of statewide injury prevention programs, was in marked contrast to other cost containment testimony the legislature had been hearing. In August 1983, cooperative efforts of the H/G-IPG with the Texas Agricultural Extension Service resulted in formulation of a call for a governor's task force on rural injury prevention. As a result of the group's activities, formal recognition and support has been forthcoming from academic institutions in Houston and Galveston. This includes the University of Texas Health Science Center at Houston, the University of Texas Medical Branch at Galveston, the Institute for Rehabilitation and Research, and the Baylor College of Medicine. The H/G-IPG also constitutes a committee of the Center for Health Promotion Research and Development at the University of Texas Health Science Center at Houston.

The H/G-IPG is working to obtain grants, mobilize public and health profession opinion, and encourage the application of proven injury prevention strategies. We believe that injury prevention education should be an integral component of medical school and other health professional curricula. A disease of such major proportion demands suitable medical education attention.

As with most serious public health problems, good intentions will not suffice for effective prevention. We believe that misinformation or misdirected efforts may be worse than doing nothing. A well-intentioned law, passed by popular demand, may be disastrous if not based on firm knowledge and without a built-in mechanism for verification of efficacy. When such laws do not accomplish the intended result, they are used as an argument against effectiveness of injury prevention legislation. Laws enabling 15- and 16-yr-old children to drive motor vehicles following completion of a driver education program may be an example [21]. Evidence suggests driver education does not safeguard these young people but may be counterproductive in allowing them to drive and hence be exposed to an increased likelihood of injury. Well-meaning but ill-conceived proposals may serve ultimately as smokescreens that hide practical solutions. For example, increased severity of punishment for driving under the influence of alcohol may appease public demand and yet be inconsequential in preventing drunk driving if not coupled with perception on the part of the drinking driver that (1) he will be apprehended, (2) punishment is certain, (3) punishment is severe, and (4) punishment is swift. This constellation of perceptions by the offender seems more important than the severity of any single one of the four [18].

While the effect of its work cannot be measured, the H/G-IPG hopes that it has helped to provide increased awareness of the injury problem and the need for effective countermeasures. Cooperative efforts between institutions and between individuals can only be beneficial in reducing serious injury and its costly consequences.

CONCLUSION

As we practice or participate in medical science, we become aware of the great changes in our society and of new worlds that unfold. As students, the old worlds of medicine were stories, rumors, and notions intermixed with science. As modern practitioners we see the real world partially with our old world eyes. We must realize that the world is in continual transition. We confront new technologies and methodologies and their associated risks and opportunities. In the area of injury prevention, we must also encourage change by expanding our visions accordingly. We must understand the moral, social, and economic aspects of injury. We can work toward new technologies, scientific insight, and information while encouraging and demanding application of currently known technologies and countermeasures to help create a world where violent death is not accepted as commonplace but as extraordinary.

REFERENCES

1. Accident facts, preliminary condensed edition. National Safety Council, March 1983.
2. The need for a national trauma institute. Position paper of the American Trauma Society, 1982.
3. Medical news. JAMA 1984;251:1645–49.
4. Baker S, O'Neill B, Karpf R. The injury fact book. Lexington, Mass.: Lexington Books, D.C. Heath & Co., 1984.

5. The highway loss reduction status report. Insurance Institute for Highway Safety 1984;19:1–12.
6. Robertson LS. Injuries: causes, control strategies and public policy. Lexington, Mass.: Lexington Books, D.C. Heath & Co., 1983.
7. The highway loss reduction status report. Insurance Institute for Highway Safety 1984;19:6.
8. Kraus JF, Black NA, Hessol N, et al. The incidence of acute brain injury and serious impairment in a defined population. Am J Epidem 1984;119:186–201.
9. Hartunian NS, Smart CN, Thompson MS. The incidence and economic costs of cancer, motor vehicle injuries, coronary heart disease, and stroke: a comparative analysis. Am J Public Health 1980;70:1249–60.
10. Iskrant AP, Joliet PV. Accidents and homicide. Cambridge, Mass.: Harvard University Press, 1968.
11. AMA Council on Scientific Affairs. Automobile related injuries: components, trends, prevention. JAMA 1983;249:3216–22.
12. Zuska JJ. Wounds without cause. Bull Am Coll Surg 1981;66:5–10.
13. Thompson CT. Alcohol and injury. Texas Med 1983;79:51–52.
14. Haddon W, Jr. Advances in the epidemiology of injuries as a basis for public policy. Public Health Rep 1980;95:411–19.
15. The highway loss reduction status report. Insurance Institute for Highway Safety. 1984;19:1–12.
16. Baker S. Medical data and injuries. Am J Public Health 1983;73:733–34.
17. Key MM. NIOSH injury surveillance system. Texas Med 1983;79:58–59.
18. Ross HL. Deterring the drinking driver: legal policy and social control. Lexington, Mass.: Lexington Books, D.C. Heath & Co., 1981.
19. Highway Loss Data Institute. Injury and collision loss experience. Washington, D.C., September 1983.
20. Report of the Conference on the Control and Prevention of Injury, Galveston, Texas, May 26–28, 1982.
21. Robertson LS. Crash involvement of teenaged drivers when drivers education is eliminated. Am J Public Health 1980;249:3216–22.

Index